Lucy Libido Says...
There's an Oil for THAT

A Girlfriend's Guide to Using
Essential Oils
Between the Sheets

Lucy Libido Says....
There's an Oil for THAT
A Girlfriend's Guide to Using
Essential Oils
Between the Sheets

ISBN – 13: 978 – 1530690794

ISBN – 10: 153069079x

Acknowledgements

While I do love my large online group of BFFs, there are special women who have humored my experiments, inspired me, cheered me on, or held my hand through the making of this book. To these friends, I thank you for being a part of something so special.

Jennifer Boyd	Emily Morrow
Heidi Bragg	Danica Nelson
Ann Estacio	Jill Noelle
Nicole Groves	Jen O'Sullivan
Sarah Harrison	Jessica Petty
Jessica King	Sarah Plunk
Kelsi Meldrum	Amy Russell
Julianna Lorenzen	Andra Smith
Deanna McMahon	Jill Ulander
Julie Sanches	Sarah Wilde

My biggest thanks goes to my bestie and accomplice, Betsy Bosom, who called me up and said "Lucy! People *need* this information. Turn it into a book already!" She believed in me, so I believed in myself.

And my gratitude would not be complete without thanking God who has blessed me with interesting and unusual gifts. Some of which are humor, articulation and unabashed flair. He has blessed me by molding me in unexpected ways to give something good to the world.

Dedication

There is a very special person who understands my heart like none other. We met when I was just 18 years old, and he waited patiently for me to grow up.

Patience is a hallmark amongst his many qualities. He recognizes my free spirit, allows me room to fly, while simultaneously being my perch, rock, and anchor.

We agreed when we were married that we would support each other in whatever individual pursuits we needed to fulfill our respective hearts. He has never wavered from this promise. Writing this book has been an exceptional testament to this. He has generously stepped up and supported me in diverse ways to give me the time and freedom to allow this book to take flight.

To you, I dedicate this book and I thank you for being my perfect eternal soul mate.

I love you... Mr. Libido

XOXO

Table of Contents

Hello

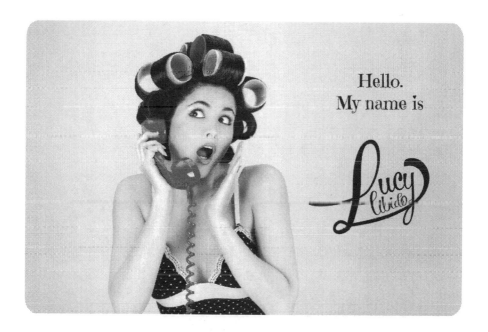

Hello.
My name is
Lucy Libido

Hello! My name is Lucy. Lucy Libido. Yup! That's my name.

Before embarking on the ***faaabulous***, that is the Lucy Libido girlfriend's guide, I want to tell you a little bit about myself.

You may have picked up this book because you are an Essential Oil lover, or perhaps because you are looking for more WOW in the bedroom. Better yet, maybe you are lucky enough to find yourself in the league of being an oil Facebook friend with a friend of a friend of a friend of Lucy. Lucky you.

Well, just in case you aren't fortunate to be a Lucy friend four times removed, you *might* have some preconceptions about this whole Lucy Libido lady. While I *am* the Venus of the modern-day oilers world, (Thank you, Thank you) the galaxy does not revolve around me. I am not flawless. I do not attract men like bees to honey only to watch them wilt in submission at the sight of my voluptuous silhouette.

Here is what you should know about me. This book has been a while in the making. A few years ago, I became an oil believer as I witnessed my young daughters barking cough dissipate before my eyes after an application of Breathe Again™ Roll-On oil. After that, I started using therapeutic grade essential oils for EVERYTHING. I used them for natural healthcare, cleaning, emotional release, courage, and even for (gasp) time spent in the bedroom.

There's not a lot written on this subject. Most of what I learned was from a friend of a friend. We would ask each other, "what do you use for this" or "what should he use for that". We would conjecture based on juicy gossip and share our little secrets with each other. I decided there was a need for a more formal libido and oils class (as formal as that can be). So, why not research and teach one myself? It could be fun to teach on ways to use oils to improve our libidos and sexuality. I also wanted it to be a place where everyone could leave having experienced a deeper connection to the person they love most. So, I created a special private Facebook group called Lucy Libido.

And in Lucy Libido, I learned a lot about myself.

And when I say that I learned a lot about myself, - I mean we learned a lot about us. You see, I am not a ME. I am a WE. Lucy is not ONE person. Lucy is a collaboration of 20 women who got together and shared:

- Our secrets
- Our tips and tools
- Our frustrations
- Our fantasies
- Our Insecurities
- Our passions
- Our failures
- Our successes

We all committed to use our essential oils in the bedroom and then to unapologetically share our results with each other. We shared what made us tick. We shared what worked for our spouses. We shared our roadblocks. We found solutions together. We cheered each other on.

Then we announced that we would be sharing our results from the Lucy Libido group in an online event. What I thought would be a small private class of yearning women turned into a phenomenon. People came in droves. Every time I turned on my computer, my inbox was full of messages, friend requests, questions, and pleas for support. It was tenfold what I had expected. I had to call in the oil squad to help authorize and approve them all. The threads grew like deep canyons. There were so many questions. So many women had issues and they wanted help. So many women who looked and sounded… well… *exactly* like Lucy.

What describes Lucy Libido? Put aside the vision of Aphrodite in all her sumptuous glory. This is what I *really* look like.

- I am in my 30's

- I am in my 40's and in my 50's and my 60's and beyond.

- I am divorced and remarried and I have a blended family.

- I am still learning what works for me in the bedroom.

- I am learning to not fight over how often is "often enough".

- I can never find time; I am too busy with the kids.

- I can't remember the last time we were intimate.

- I have pain - I'm working towards enjoying intercourse.

- I am in my 20's

- I have spent considerable time in multiple relationships, looking for the right one.

- I married young to the first man who asked and I have never known another.

- I am too exhausted for sex.

- I want romance more but my husband is seldom home.

- I lost the drive after childbirth and I want it back.

- I can remember the last time but I'm confused if it's "good enough".

- I feel "broken". I struggle to climax.
- I feel like I can't keep up with my husband's sexual appetite.
- My hormones stopped working after childbirth/surgery/medications/disease.
- He needs some help in the firmness department.
- He will not let me touch him with the oils. (Yet....)
- I don't feel "sexy" enough.
- I am navigating around a big 'ol pregnant belly right now.
- I'm confused because I always want it, and he rarely does.
- I need some help in the libido department.
- He seems to finish right when I get started.
- I just want to **want** it again

I am short, tall, thin, wide, curvy, square, and downright human. I am pretty much, well, just like you. If you found a phrase up there that sounds familiar – rest assured that we are going to be friends. And not like a friend of a friend of a friend. A *real* girlfriend. The kind that's been there, has shared her vulnerabilities and has a little guidance for ya. So, no matter what category you find yourself in, sit back, relax, roll on a little Lavender, take a big whiff and slowly exhale. This is going to be fun. After all, you are just like "me".

Or at least *one* of me.

XOXO

Hello

Beautiful

Lucy Libido

Now that you know a little about me, it's time to get to know a little about you. So, go grab a pen. Do you have a cute pen you love? Awesome! Time to wield it like a boss. Got colors? Choose turquoise or pink—I mean if you are artistic enough to have colored pens on hand, then you should definitely color coordinate with the cover, no doubt. Get ready to jot down a few notes for me. I know, I know. You probably weren't expecting a book titled "Lucy Libido" to be extremely introspective, but this is very important. Consider it your initiation to being an *official* BFF of Lucy.

This book is all about oils and libido. (You got that from the cover I presume). Well, before we even talk oils, you need to know that a big part of feeling sexy is not defined by how you look physically. It comes from an inner panache that emanates from the core moving outward. It's a silent but seductive confidence of *knowing* that You-Are-Beautiful.

One of the things a lot of my friends told me is that they don't feel "sexy enough". Most of them have bodies that have changed with time. Their silhouettes have transitioned through pregnancy, time, age or injury. Perhaps they never deemed themselves "sexy enough" to start with; viewing themselves as replete with cosmetic flaws or lacking in virtues to self-love. "Sexy enough" is subjective. If the definition of sexy is tall and thin with huge doll-like eyes, then I'm toast. If it's pore-less skin, no wrinkles, collar bone-hugging cleavage and a two-inch gap between the thighs... then, yeah. *None* of us are sexy, myself included.

But, listen here. That is not what dictates sexy. That is not what defines beauty. I asked my cohorts of Lucy friends to tell me what makes them beautiful. What makes them wonderful? What makes them, *sexy*? I asked them to describe what makes their spouses attracted to them.

You know what--they had a **hard** time. They had a hard time describing what makes them beautiful, especially, beyond their physical features. Most of them did not answer. I think that was a wakeup call.

I think that we are so focused on our so-called "flaws" that we forget to embrace everything that is beautiful about ourselves. And do you know what the MOST beautiful and sexy thing is????? A woman who **knows** that she is beautiful!

I think we need to be a little kinder; a little more self-forgiving. I remember a day when I was putting on a swimsuit and my hips hadn't seen the sun in many months. The paleness of my trunk made the light faint streaks of my stretch marks that were usually unnoticeable a bit more prominent. I heard two voices, one speaking in each ear. The critical voice impulsively said, *"You can see them. Everyone will see them"*. But the forgiving voice was so much more kind. She said, *"Let the whole world see. For they are your badges of grace and honor; to be worn with pride. They represent the greatest pain you ever endured, to bring to pass the greatest joy you've ever known."*

We wake up every day and balance these voices. The critical voice is not necessarily shallow, nor is she bad. She knows that when I find clothes that fit me well – I feel better about how I look. She knows that when I physically prepare myself for the day, I am more productive. She knows that when I take the time to look my best, then I also feel my best. She knows that when I see beauty in myself, then I see it in others.

But the forgiving voice is important too. She is a little quieter and too often muffled by the constant noise of life. She is a little more reverent, poised, and a lot more wise. She reminds me of my strength. She is vital because she emphasizes my value.

If you have parts of your body that you don't love, rest assured, you're not alone. Welcome to the ever popular I-don't-love-my _____(fill in the blank)_____ club. Some features you may be able to ameliorate with your own efforts and in doing so, you may find more confidence and happiness. Good for you. Other features may not be so easily improved, or don't hold much value in changing, and perhaps those you should only look at with love and amnesty. Let those go. The way you express and value beauty can be individual. If you dislike a scar, you are not wrong or overly vain for not embracing it like the woman next door. Likewise, if the woman next door does little to improve a scar, she is not wrong for being overly lazy or careless.

You are going to hear the critical voice and the forgiving voice. Just know that they are not bad and that they are both an important part of you. Balance them with aplomb. But, if you hear a voice that tells you that you aren't beautiful enough, or sexy enough or *good* enough to be with a partner – be aware that you are no longer listening to something that is a part of you. You are listening to outright *lies* because you ARE enough and your beauty is inextricably bonded to your name.

I love these pictures. To me, they represent beauty in its multiple 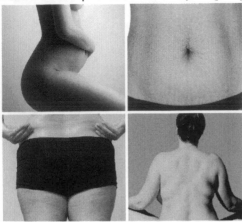 forms. They show courage and strength and authenticity. They are real bodies. They are beautiful bodies. They are bodies just like Lucy and her friends, and probably yours. They are beautiful! Whether you are short, tall, thin, curvy, plump, frail, nipped/tucked, saggy, scarred, stretched, petite, plus, muscular, soft, voluptuous, or taut, you are BEAUTIFUL!

Ok. Pick up your pen. It's time for initiation. This is your challenge. On the top line, I've already written: "I am BEAUTIFUL." On the following lines, write down the hallmarks of your own unique beauty. Think of the attributes you are proud to possess. Notate the stunning facets that make you proud to be YOU. Or, describe the beauty that others see in you. If you need some help, here are some ideas from my friends when we did this together.

- I'm beautiful because I can laugh at anything.
- I see beauty in my hips that have grown each time I grew our little ones.
- He cherishes the little noise I make when he kisses my neck.
- My beauty is my boldness – I surprise him with something sexy under a nightshirt.
- My beauties are my eyes and my quick wit.
- My spouse sees beauty in my peculiarities; he loves the way I run up the stairs on my toes.
- My significant other loves my hair, my curves, and my goofiness.
- My ability to give is what makes me beautiful.

I Am Beautiful!

_____

_____

_____

_____

_____

_____

_____

_____

_____

_____

_____

_____

_____

_____

_____

_____

Good job! That wasn't TOO hard, was it? (Girlfriend you'd better not be reading this unless that page is filled out). Now you are **officially** one of my BFFs! Congrats! Now that you've filled out the many ways that you are beautiful; I want you to revisit them every time you pick up this book. I want you to literally open to this page first, and remind yourself what makes you awesome, unique and individually beautiful. You'll probably have more come to mind in the next few days, and I want you to add them as you go. There's space in the back for more thoughts as needed.

Remind your critical voice that there's a place here for her too. She knows that you are amazing, but she still wants to put her best self forward. Well, never fear. In our recipe section, I have listed some tried and true recipes for fading stretch marks, diminishing leg veins and smoothing dimpled skin. (Friends don't let friends have lingering stretch marks when you have a secret recipe to help them fade.) There are even recipes to help him put *his* best "foot" forward. One nice, solid, sturdy foot…

Last thing: Friend to friend. Do me a favor. If you are reading this, please join with all my other BFFs. Get a piece of paper. Write on it "I am Beautiful". Take a selfie while holding your paper. Email it to Betsy at betsybosom@lucylibido.com. We'll post it on the Lucy Libido Blog. Then, come find your picture at www.lucylibido.com.

I believe that you are wonderful. You are exquisite. You are discerning and critical, but forgiving. You are beautiful. Say it to yourself once in a while.

The more you say it – the more you will believe it. The more you believe it – the more you will know it. The more you know it, the more you will own in. And when you OWN it GIRL………..

That's when you become a Lucy Libido.

XOXO

Lucy

How to use

Aphrodisiac
oils

OK, let's talk really quick about where to get and how to use your oils. I know you must be super excited to discover the best oils for him and her. But first, I want to make sure that you are using them safely. Therapeutic grade essential oils are *very* potent. It takes 150 pounds of lavender blossoms to make 1lb of pure therapeutic grade lavender oil. For this reason, a 100% pure and therapeutic grade lavender will be of more value than one that is cut with lavandin (a hybrid plant that has a similar smell to lavender but is cheaper) or oils that are pre-diluted with carrier oil or are altogether synthetic.

A true essential oil is the lifeblood of the plant. Oils carry valuable properties inherent to the plant. Each plant has a different value based on its chemical makeup. When taken from the plant and used in the human body, this lifeblood bestows those same properties into the human body. It's crazy cool. These properties are called chemical constituents and they are what make essential oils living, bioavailable superstars.

Take Cypress for example. Cypress is one of my FAVORITE oils. So much so, that whenever it goes out of stock at Young Living, my friends all tease me that I must have recently bought up *all* the Cypress in bulk. I always get the wrap for Cypress going out of stock. It's sad and only sometimes true. Can't a girl love her Cypress? Sheesh!

Cypress is high in Alpha-Pinene, which falls in a group of chemical constituents called monoterpenes. Monoterpenes work in the body to inhibit the accumulation of toxins and help discharge existing toxins from the liver and kidney. In Cypress, there are antiseptic, expectorant and diuretic qualities.

Cypress is a fantastic support to the circulatory system. It is naturally hemostatic and styptic; which means that it strengthens the blood vessel walls and aids them to close in the case of an open cut or wound. The naturally occurring camphene is also antiseptic which means it acts against bacteria and reduces the chance of infection. So, when there is any kind of injury to the body, cypress can help to support the body's natural defenses to stop bleeding and prevent infection. Even cooler though, is how these same properties work to improve circulation when the blood vessels have not been broken.

Cypress has long been known to strengthen blood vessels by increasing their ability to contract and release, which improves blood flow. Weak vein walls coupled with improper circulatory pressure can make blood pool in veins causing them to stretch and widen or bulge towards the surface. This can result in varicose or spider veins. When applied daily to these large or spidery veins, Cypress improves the vein's ability to push the blockage of blood that makes them appear raised and dark. Thus, making leg veins appear smaller, lighter and less noticeable (Recipe at the back).

Cypress is also a gentle diuretic; which means it aids in flushing out toxins. This is why Cypress is one of the main ingredients in Cell-Lite massage oil, a fantastic naturally derived tushytoning massage oil. Dimpled backsides are no girl's favorite and can sometimes be caused by fluid retention, lack of circulation, a breakdown of collagen, fibrous tissues, and excess body fat. Even thin girlies lose tone over time. Cypress helps reduce the appearance of cellulite by reducing excess fluid, improving blood flow and increasing toxin removal during urination.

While we're talking about it, Grapefruit is the other therapeutic superstar in Cell-lite massage oil. Grapefruit is high in D-limonene. D-limonene[1] aids in lipolysis[2]; which is the process of breaking down fats and releasing them into the bloodstream to be used as energy (known as ketones). Excess ketones and toxins are also flushed out through your liver and excreted through urine. This is where Cypress and Grapefruit work so-well together – the Grapefruit helps to break down fatty tissue, and Cypress helps to strengthen the circulation and helps flush out excess toxins and ketones.

Amazing, right? It makes my bootay look better, my legs look better, it makes my chest feel clearer and it's relaxing in a diffuser. Try it in the diffuser with Lavender. AHHHH! Sooooo many reasons to love Cypress. And I haven't even *gotten* to how to use Cypress between the sheets. That's another chapter. But, all this is to say, that therapeutic chemical constituents in essential oils have the ability to improve, repair and restore our bodies to function at their best. And such results only occur when you are using a Therapeutic Grade Essential Oil.

I'll be honest when I say that I've been around the block. I don't mean around the block with men. I'm a strictly monogamous gal. I mean I've been around the block with oils. I have tried all the brands. The big brands, and the little brands. The "scientific" brands, and the online brands. The health-food store brands, and the cheap bulk brands. I have learned that quality matters.

1 limonene http://www.ncbi.nlm.nih.gov/pubmed/16637681

2 lipolysis and grapefruit - http://www.ncbi.nlm.nih.gov/pubmed/15862904

Cut-rate oils are inexpensive because they either only contain a small amount of essential oil (but can still legally be labeled as pure) or the oil is a lower quality fragrance grade oil. Fragrance grade oils still come from the plant, but do not contain medicinal value. Chemical constituents are very sensitive and can generally only be extracted through low heat and pressure. Ramping up the heat, pressure, or extracting with solvents will pull more oil out of the plant giving greater volume, but at the cost of killing the molecules that work in our body therapeutically.

Personally, I only use Therapeutic Grade oils now that are grown, distilled, tested and sealed with a Seed to Seal guarantee. I'm not sponsored to say so; it's what I trust. Young Living is the only company that farms and distills their own oils themselves. Unlike every other brand, they are *not* a middleman who buys from other sources to rebottle, rebrand and then resell. I like knowing that they own or co-op their farms. They grow their flowers, plants, and trees without harmful pesticides. They test with higher standards than any other company, and they ship them from the farm to your door. There is an abundance of chemical laden oils that are labeled as pure. Adulterating oils with unlabeled carrier oil is almost the norm among cheaper brands. You will not get the constituent benefits of therapeutic grade cypress or grapefruit when using cut-rate oil. You just won't. Lucy and her friends will not be held responsible if you get sick from ingesting synthetic oil. And we'll wave the I-told-you-so finger if you break out in a rash after putting cheap oils with hidden alcohol solvents near your lady bits. And believe me when I say that this has happened, and it will definitely NOT improve your libido.

Here is how you can use your Young Living Aphrodisiac Oils:

Aromatic

Get yourself a diffuser. If you have a premium starter kit, BRAVO! You already have a medical grade high quality diffuser. Use your oil of choice and put 5-8 drops in your diffuser with filtered water. Tap water will work too, but the minerals will wear your diffuser out faster.

Diffusing aphrodisiac oils disperses them into the air to be inhaled. Not only do they smell wonderful, they directly impact your brain in a fascinating way. Love, peace, sensuality, and calm are all emotions that can be triggered by oils. Your brain is composed of several parts, but to keep it simple, we have a "thinking brain" (your frontal cortex) and your "feeling/emotional brain" (your limbic brain). Your frontal cortex is logical, analytical, and is used to solve problems. The limbic area of the brain is where our emotions lie. Feelings such as happiness, sadness, anxiety or peace, anger or love, all emanate from this region; so do impulses such as hunger and thirst, and sexual desire.

Essential oils can have a profound effect on your mood because they are unique in that they get past that "thinking brain" and impact your "feeling brain". When you inhale essential oil molecules, the olfactory bulb triggers the limbic area of the brain. It stimulates the amygdala, which is the center for our sexual drive. They also have been shown to stimulate the hippocampus, which is responsible for memory. Oils with sesquiterpene molecules are so tiny that they can even cross the blood-brain barrier and oxygenate the pineal gland which is associated with the regulation of hormones and spiritual attunement. Diffusing Essential Oils sends signals to the brain to relax and enjoy. This can help usher in the mood, or help with frigidity. There are particular oils that tend to do this the most. But, don't worry too much about choosing the "right" oils. There are mood enhancing diffuser recipes at the back, but much of it will be what you prefer. There is no right or wrong. Choose what you enjoy.

Topical

Apply your oils topically. You can apply in several locations. If you are familiar with Vitaflex points, you can apply oils to the Vitaflex points for male and female reproductive systems. The point for female reproduction is the outer right ankle. The Vitaflex point for the brain is the thumb of the hand and big toe of the foot. For the male, his reproductive Vitaflex point is his outer left ankle. Don't stress this one too much. If you (a woman) accidentally put oils on the outside of your left ankle - I promise it won't hurt you and you won't start growing a beard. More common places to apply topically are the chest, behind the neck, the forehead, behind the ears, on the wrists, or below the navel. For oils to stimulate erogenous zones, you apply the oils on the inner thighs from the mid-thigh up to the panty line, and/or below the navel. Apply them on the inner thigh from the mid-thigh all the way up into the panty crease. This is an especially good place for oils that boost hormones, increase circulation, or promote lubrication. This goes for women OR men.

Any time you are using oil for the first time, you should dilute it in half in carrier oil (one drop EO in one drop grapeseed oil, for example) and apply it to the forearms. It is extremely rare to have an allergy, intolerance, or hypersensitivity to an oil. But while it is rare, it is not impossible. Diluting and applying on the forearm is a safe way to assess the reaction of your skin with any particular oil. We're going to learn more later about using oils for his and her sensual massage. Yup! We've got recipes. OH, do we have recipes. Again – dilute and test on your forearm first. Lucy is not responsible for crispy burned Yayas or deflated Hoses if you don't heed to my wisdom.

Never use hot oils like Thieves, Lemongrass, Peppermint, Panaway, neat (undiluted) on sensitive membranes. Hot oils should always be diluted even on regular skin. To hammer this point into your brain, I'm going to share a little story.

"Once upon a time, there was a woman named Lucy. She was a pro at diluting EO's into carrier oils for bedroom fun. She always tried new oils on her arm first and diluted when using oils on sensitive areas.

One day, Lucy had a bit of a headache. The night was still young, so she applied peppermint to her head to ease the tension and made for a more enjoyable night. She was changing into something cute and was too lazy to go out and grab her regular diluted bedroom-time blends.

For some crazy reason, she used the peppermint she had on her hand, and wiped a drop onto her lady parts for lubrication.

She screamed in sheer terror as it burned her poor little lady bits to kingdom come. She hopped with knees crossed like a lame rabbit to the kitchen to retrieve grapeseed oil for a rinse. There was no amount of carrier oil in the world that could get it off fast enough, and the night was OFFICIALLY over."

The end.

Now you'll always remember.

Internal Use of Essential Oils

We're almost at the fun, fun, oil-me-up part. But first, let's clear up some questions that a lot of people have about ingesting oils.

Young Living Essential Oil are distilled and bottled so that if the plant is edible, then the oil is edible. This is one thing that sets them apart from any other copycat company in the world.

Lemon is an edible plant. Therefore, lemon oil is an edible oil. So long as it is not distilled with chemicals, solvents, or blended with synthetic fragrances (very common with over the counter oils), then it is edible. It absorbs into your stomach and aids the liver in producing glutathione, which is responsible for removing toxins from the body. It's pretty cool.

There are many oils that may surprise you that are edible too! Like Bergamot comes from the citrus family like lemon. Frankincense and Lavender are edible. Idaho Blue Spruce, Goldenrod, and Nutmeg are generally regarded as safe for internal consumption (Also known as GRAS).

Young Living just made labeling easier for using oils internally. They have a line of oils called Vitality. You will recognize them by their white labels. All the Vitality oils have instructions for internal use right on the label just like you would see with a vitamin. Easy!

If the oil comes in the Vitality line, then it's safe for ingestion. But, not every ingestible oil is in the line yet. As of this writing, Copaiba, Idaho Blue Spruce, Goldenrod, Nutmeg are a few examples of oils that are regarded safe for consumption but are not yet in the Vitality line. You should always check on proper application methods in your Desk Reference or your Reference Guide for Essential Oils.

The Desk Reference of the Reference Guide both gives clear and easy instructions on application methods of *all* oils. If an oil is regarded as safe for consumption, then it will list oral directions for use as a dietary supplement.

When in doubt – all Young Living oils may be used aromatically or topically when properly diluted. But, if you are already comfortable with your oils or you would like to learn how to use them systemically via ingestion as a dietary supplement, then follow the directions for dietary supplementation in these reference guides. There is also a simple reference chart in the back that shows which Lucy Libido oils are appropriate for internal use.

One of the benefits of ingesting oils is that they can work directly with the digestive system; they work systemically through the body to aid in releasing toxins and to support healthy hormonal balance. Healthy hormones are happy hormones and you want your hormones to be as chipper as they can be.

Just as you would dilute a new oil that you apply topically, you always want to dilute any new oil you use internally as well. I've come to find that my body is fine with citrus oils with no dilution needed. However hot oils like peppermint, oregano, and Thieves are absorbed more comfortably when I use them in a clear empty capsule filled with several drops of olive oil. This is the case with most people. As a good rule of thumb, I recommend you try a new oil topically before you use it internally. Also, when consuming an essential oil for the first time, you should always dilute that essential oil in olive oil.

One of my favorite recipes for him is an internal capsule that may be able to replace a convenient little hexagonal tablet that he's been taking. It works by improving circulation, blood flow, and increasing testosterone levels. Just keep turning the pages my friend; keeeeep on turning. It's about to get warm in here.

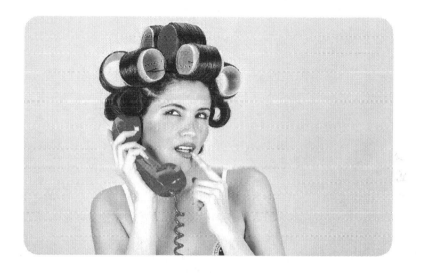

The Libido Seesaw

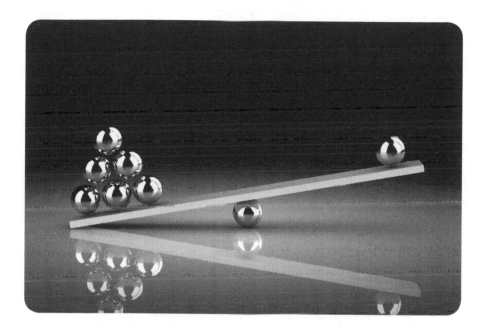

Let's chat a little bit about the libido seesaw. Many loyal couples find themselves frustrated in their relationships. Not because of unfaithfulness, but for a lack of spark and desire. The most common reasons that loyal couples seek out professional assistance are: lack of libido, difficulty climaxing or performing, decline in frequency after childbirth or life changes, and mismatched sex drives.

I want you to think about the person you love. I want you to envision yourself with that person next to a seesaw. In front of that seesaw is a large container full of large round silver balls. Now, I want both you and your loved one to grab a burlap sack. That sack has a big ol' honest word across it. That word is "Libido".

I want you to both fill your sack with the amount of silver balls that correspond to your individual libidos. Now, go put it on the seesaw. What do you see?

If you are like many couples – one side will probably tip down and the other will probably tip up. It is more common for the man's side to be heavier, pressing down while the woman's side is lighter. But this is not always the case. Each relationship is unique. Regardless of who is up, and who is down, heavily mismatched sex drives can be frustrating for *both* partners.

Many times, the person who has a lighter "Libido" burlap sack doesn't necessarily *want* to have a smaller sack. Sometimes, there is just less of a need. Sometimes, medications or life's stress is impeding on a sack that may otherwise be fuller. Sometimes they want to have more desire, but he/she just doesn't know how to *want to want it.*

The person with the heavier sack may feel frustration. They want to express love to the person who is their everything. They need more connection, more frequency, and more passion. They may feel torn because they want to meet these needs without causing pressure to the person on the other side of the seesaw, or without feeling constant rejection.

There was a life period when Mr. Libido and I had a very unbalanced seesaw. Part of the problem was that we were both working so much that we failed to make intimacy (or basic one-on-one time) a priority. I was also so afraid to become pregnant that it became a psychological block for me. So, I used an injected birth control that I felt was the "safest" to prevent pregnancy. But the side effect from the high levels of hormones was such that it completely destroyed my libido. To the point, that sex sounded annoying rather than enjoyable. I always felt prodded and expected, and he always felt longing and rejection. We look back and see that this particular form of birth control worked not because it prevented ovulation or implantation. Oh no, it worked primarily because we almost NEVER had sex.

Our seesaw was so unbalanced that it affected our marriage. This was a time that we fought more often, we used work as a way to escape home and we almost forgot that we chose to marry each other because we fell in love when we were best friends.

Your seesaw will rock up and down a bit. The person with the heavier sack may switch sides from time to time as well. That's natural and normal. But having one on the floor and the other in the air is not healthy. When your seesaw is more balanced, both you and your best friend on the other side will draw closer to each other. You will see less of each other's faults and more of their beauty. Your love will grow stronger as you spend more time together giving of yourself in the most beautiful way to the person you love the most.

Pulling together my BFFs and sharing what oils helped us to fill our burlap Libido sacks was initially for a small group of women. As I have watched it grow to a large online presence and even a book, I realize how very, very many unbalanced seesaws are out there. And with the gift of oils I have seen women fill their sacks, balance their seesaws, and have a higher quality of life.

What about decreasing libido in the heavy burlap sack? "Are there oils to reduce libido?" "Would that help the seesaw?" Some have asked this. Yes, there are oils that can help calm an overactive sex-drive. Camphor has been traditionally used by monks to reduce desire and keep them chaste. Marjoram has been shown in studies to reduce libido in rats.[3] But unless there is a medically overactive situation or an addiction that requires suppression, the best way to balance the seesaw is to fill the sack that is lighter.

Filling the sack that is lighter with tools to increase desire and improve fireworks will naturally lead to wanting more. Wanting more will increase frequency which tends to allow couples to be more relaxed and creative, which leads to new discoveries, passions

---

3 Marjoram and sperm count, sperm mobility, and libido in rats
  http://onlinelibrary.wiley.com/doi/10.1111/j.1742-7835.2007.00125.x/full

and more desire. As the lighter libido sack finds way to improve his/her desires, the heavier sack receives fulfillment. This doesn't necessarily "remove" libido from that person's sack, but it fills the need from which the desire stems, naturally balancing the seesaw to a place where both sides are happy and fulfilled.

Get ready to have a smile on your face next weekend because Lucy is one of your BFFs. I'm going to teach you what we learned during our "research". I'll share what helped us get in the mindset of yearning. We'll show you which oils will help you feel SO happy and fulfilled that you'll be excited for more. By the time we were done, we had a lot of balanced seesaws. This meant a lot of happy Lucys, and a lot of content Mr. Libidos.

Get Ready
Get set
to g-OOOOOO

Let's chat a bit about emotional and mental preparation. I'm like most women, and for us, sex starts way before we walk into the bedroom. Unlike men who can become aroused just by seeing their Lucy step out of the shower, we do well with a little bit of pampering and preparation. In our Lucy group, we experimented with ways to get us in the mindset of va-va-voom. We found that when we made intentional preparations during the day, we were much more likely to "find time" in the evening or not be too tired to Tango by the weekend.

I know that sometimes it's easier said than done. If you have a house full of little messmakers- oops I mean little curious minds- then you may be lucky to brush your teeth before you stage an intervention to keep your phone out of the toilet. If you are crazy busy with work, you may feel lucky to eat lunch, let alone meet up for lunch. Sometimes, it's the little things you can sneak into your day amongst that overloaded plate of life.

Think of the little steps you can take to feel sexy despite all the obstacles. Do you feel sexy when you put on a fresh face of make-up? Well, if your life dictates that you can't do that until after the kids are down, by all means, do it then. It won't be a waste being on for just a couple of hours if that means it helps you feel romantic when the house is quiet. One thing that helps build anticipation for me is taking the extra 5 minutes in the shower to shave my legs and "Lucy territory". Yes, it may mean an extra episode of cartoons for the kids but that's time well spent when it makes me feel excited that I have something fabulous coming. Here are a few other tips we found helpful.

Have a special EO infused soap that you pamper yourself with just before game time. The scent will remind you of intimacy and can invite feelings of excitement. Likewise, you can do this with a special diffuser blend. You can choose one or two blends that you diffuse just during your time together. The sense of smell can trigger anticipation for you, and it will certainly pique his interest when he walks in the room. "Honey is that the "Charm-the-Snake" blend I smell???" (You can name it whatever you want….)

Set aside time for intimacy. Yes, it may sound a little odd, almost like you're scheduling it in next to your teen's orthodontist appointment or your next pap smear. But truly, as much as spontaneity is deliciously exuberant, unless both you and your honey have lots of spare time on your hands, you are unlikely to use those hands on each other. Plan one-on-one with each other. Date your spouse. Get a sitter or create a babysitting swap with other couples. Reserve time to be alone together to reconnect and initiate intimacy.

Buy yourself some pretty panties. Yes, I said *pretty*. Wearing something pretty doesn't mean that you are less strong, doomed to submission, or inferior. You can still wear pretty lace panties and be on top whenever you wish. Whether you choose black mesh or pink lace is up to you. But putting on something that makes you look sexy will probably help you to feel sexy – and feeling sexy is the first step to being in a hungry mindset. Here's a thought. If you know you are trying to set aside time that night to be alone, start the day off by wearing something incredibly non-practical and sensual underneath. Even if you are in leggings and a T-shirt, there's something about knowing you have a lacy surprise waiting to be discovered underneath. Or, if you want to be even more of a vixen, go without panties all together. Then text Mr. Libido and tell him you are commando and time his record-speed commute home. That's a fun game.

Text him a suggestive thought or picture. "I'm wearing something teeny tiny under my dress, can you guess what it is? Maybe when I get home you'll find out….." This type of mental foreplay is extremely effective. It rouses both him and her to be aching for each other until they can meet up. A note on sexting however: it's fun but be smart about it. Always ensure that he has his phone in his hand first. Do you want to send a picture only to find out he was grabbing drinks for his team and that gnarly photo popped up on his desk in front of his clients?? EEeeehhhhhhhsshhh. Then the rule of banter is delete delete delete! If you're going to play this way, **both** of you have to know to delete both the conversation *and* the photo stream. There's nothing worse than your kids picking up your phone to text daddy and seeing HELLO MOMMY in the prior message. Oh wait. Actually, there is something worse. It's worse when you are scrolling through your photo stream with a mom from pre-school to show her your kid's talent show pictures and you scroll into "come-home-honey" pictures that you forgot to remove. OH MY GOSH.

Once in a while, treat yourself to something that you want. It can be a pair of jeans that flatter your hips and you had to save for. Many of my friends mentioned a splurge for a haircut, massage, or facial. Maybe it is a few hours with a personal trainer. We all have different wish lists. Without a doubt there is never enough funds for everything on our wish lists all at once. Still, allowing the kindness of gifting to ourselves in moderation has value. We are demonstrating to ourselves that we are deserving of something that brings us happiness.

Use your oils to de-stress. There are days when you feel like you might want to pull your hair out. Remember that oils are unique in that they can cross the blood brain barrier and oxygenate the part of your brain that deals with emotions. Diffuse some Peace and Calming or Joy to keep your "I'm-going-crazy meter" at or below maniac. Apply Stress Away or Tranquil so you don't want to kill your spouse over minor offenses like not changing the empty toilet paper roll. (This never happens at our house). Diffuse the sleep inducing oils to get kids down to bed early. Then oil yourself up with heart-pumping, lube-secreting, desire-enhancing, leg-crossing aphrodisiac oils, and saunter your way into his arms and give him a big molten kiss.

Progessence Plus™

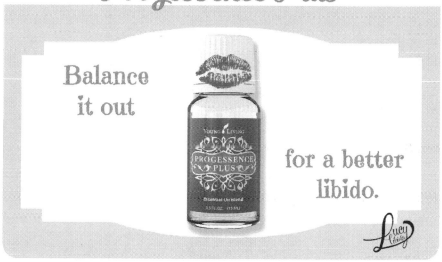

Balance it out

for a better libido.

It happens every month. It's like there's some kind of *cycle* to it. Not only do I notice the change.... but my body does too. It tells me that I need Progessence Plus. So I use it and of course then Mr. Libido gets to hear about it. This is a recurring conversation with Mr. Libido.

- "Have I told you how GREAT Progessence Plus is?"
- "Yes. You told me about 28 days ago."
- "My head has totally stopped pounding"
- "You said that 56 days ago"
- "I feel sooooooo much better now! I don't have to sleep all day"
- "You mentioned that 84 days ago".

I have this repeating cycle of talking non-stop about how much I LOVE Progessence Plus. I tend to talk a lot about it, in fact, every 28 days or so.

A few years ago, and after my third baby, I started getting Migraines. They would keep me in bed with my eyes covered. The only way I could function on those days were sleeping for hours during the day while the kids were at school, and then taking caffeine and painkillers to get me through the afternoon. I remember one day I had to take my baby into daycare just so I could sleep in a dark room, it was so bad. They didn't happen every day, maybe once a month. It would last a day or two and then disappear.

I was on a trip once when I felt the throbbing starting on the sides of my head. A good friend of mine, who was also a nurse, was sharing a hotel room with me. She was also an "oiler". Noticing my bathroom clutter, she said "That's a menstrual migraine, Lucy. Do you have some Progessence?"

Now LUCY is the kind of person who would never NEED Progessence. NOOOOO, that's just for women with endometriosis or severe PMS. I am the love queen. I am happy all the time, not subject to irritability ever, and am 100% sexy day and night. Even on my period, I smell of roses and hummingbirds flutter about my head.

"Nah, I'm just overtired." I said, and popped my pill.

About a month later – it started again. I kinda noticed something this time…. It was about a month since my last migraine. Hmmmmm. So, I ordered the hormone balancing oil that is supposed to help everything from libido to migraines. I figured it would be good to have it on hand.

Then AGAIN. A month later – I felt it returned. Like clockwork.

Then I learned how unbalanced I really was. And how much happier I would become knowing how to balance hormones with natural plant extracts.

Life is all about balance. We balance our professional and private lives. We balance our proteins and carbs. We balance home life with work life. It's all a balancing act! In yoga, there's a pose called Scorpion, where you're balancing on your arms and your body is arched over the head, like a scorpion stinger. A person needs 100% balance and focus to achieve that pose! If your core isn't activated, if your arms aren't supported, if your legs are too far forward, it's just not going to happen. It's VERY much the same with our hormones and libido.

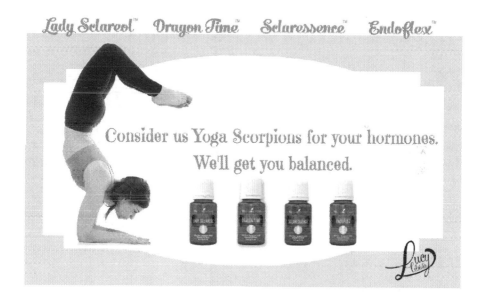

Lady Sclareol™ Dragon Time™ Sclaressence™ EndoFlex™

Consider us Yoga Scorpions for your hormones. We'll get you balanced.

Here's a story from one of my BFFs.

I knew for years that my hormones were out of balance. Several babies in a short amount of time coupled with intense stress and a poor diet affected most areas of my life. I was feeling sluggish, crabby, and definitely not sexy or beautiful! I had no desire for sexual intimacy and would often pretend like I was asleep so my husband wouldn't get any ideas.

Bless Mr. Libido, he was so very understanding, but he has needs too and that made me feel even more inadequate because I wasn't able to meet them. Several years ago when I realized I was crazy out of whack, I was just starting out on my personal journey to a healthier lifestyle, so I wanted to find a natural way to put my body back into its natural balance. Makes sense, right?

Fast forward about a year later, and I discovered essential oils. Cool! Then I hear about Progessence Plus Serum. Even cooler! It's not an essential oil, but a natural progesterone supplement with essential oils and wild yam extract. The first time I tried it, I felt nothing different. But I was much nicer to my kids! The second time I tried it... let's just say that I'm glad my husband works from home, and I'm glad we have a lock on our bedroom door! Mr. Libido was so happy that I'd found something that helped me get frisky. I had my sex drive back!! It was definitely an unexpected outcome, but a very nice one!

This isn't a "quick fix" supplement, but for me in the long term, it has helped reset my hormonal balance and given that part of my life back.

Progessence Plus was developed by a Doctor who specializes in women's hormonal issues. When testing women who came to see him, almost all of them had low progesterone or ZERO progesterone. This is a problem, because this is a hormone that our body needs in adequate amounts for our libido and overall

These statements have not been evaluated by the Food and Drug Administration. Products discussed are not intended to diagnose, treat, cure, or prevent any disease

wellness. Many women's issues like endometriosis, menstrual migraines, and PMS may be related to low levels of natural progesterone. Low progesterone and/or estrogen also contribute to hot flashes and night sweats. Progesterone production decreases over time and tends to drop after childbirth for many women. When it drops too low, our sex drive disappears too. Boo!

Well, the next time my head started pounding, I followed the advice of my friends. I applied Progessence Plus to my forearms and the back of my neck. I drank lots of water and Ninxia Zyng with a touch of caffeine. To my utter delight, the pounding dissipated. And every 28 days or so when I start to feel it creeping in, I know my body's levels are too low. I found that low progesterone presents differently in different bodies which is why it affects libido in one, PMS in another, and migraines in the next. So, whenever any of my friends is dealing with any of these things, I tell them to try Progessence Plus first. And now, at least once a month, it becomes my best friend and Mr. Libido gets to hear alllllll about it.

Besides Progessence Plus, there are a few other hormone balancing oils you should know about. Lady Sclareol and Sclaressence are Essential Oils blends that also work to balance the female reproductive system. These blends both increase and support healthy estradiol levels. Estradiol supports the ovaries and uterus for reproductive purposes and it supports the bones and joints lifelong. Estradiol levels drop with age and especially so for some during menopause. Women who have naturally higher estradiol levels tend to have fewer issues with fertility and have more substantial bone mass.[4]

Natural hormones abound in our body and are necessary for reproduction and other vital systems. Phytoestrogens, like those found in Clary Sage are plant hormones that are similar to mammal estrogens and are bioavailable in the body. Cool eh?!

---

4 Estrogen and bone mass - - http://www.ncbi.nlm.nih.gov/pubmed/8865143

However, synthetic progesterone and synthetic estrogen are NOT completely compatible with the body. The incompatibility and synthetic nature of these products are such that they have serious side effects.... and serious means B.A.D. Like a-disease-we-shall-not-name bad.

When the body has high levels of natural hormones, either from human or plant derived hormones, the risks of said diseases DECREASED. When the body has low levels of natural hormones, or is pumped with synthetic hormones, the risks of these diseases INCREASED.[5]

Moral of the study:

- Human hormones. GOOD.
- Plant hormones. OKAY.
- Synthetic hormones? BAD.

Lady Sclareol and Sclaressence

Lady Sclareol is for topical use and can be used as needed to improve mood and wellness as it can be used daily for hormone support. It can be worn as a perfume and some swear it works better when applied by their male partner. Sclaressence is a special blend of oils that are ingestible and can be used as a dietary supplement to support hormone balance and the female reproductive system.

Dragon Time

Dragon Time is a hormone balancing oil that was developed JUST for that time of the month. Ahhhhhh yup. That "Dragon Time". It contains a blend of oils that help to ease cramped

5 Disease rates among progesterone deficient women - http://www.ncbi.nlm.nih.gov/pubmed/7304556

muscles, improve mood, calm the mind and balance hormones. It helps to tame the dragon. I love it in a hot Epsom bath. This one is gentle enough that even teens can use it. Don't you wish you had this when you were a teenager?

Endoflex

Endoflex is an endocrine supporting blend. The endocrine system is responsible for telling your body what hormones to produce and when to produce them. It regulates metabolism, growth and development, tissue function, sexual function, reproduction, sleep and mood. Endoflex supports the pineal and pituitary glands and adrenal glands.

Using Endoflex daily can support overall endocrine health. This can be beneficial for the thyroid, for metabolism, and for energy. It can even benefit libido as part of a total package of hormonal balance. Endoflex essential oil can be used topically over the thyroid, kidneys, or liver and Endoflex Vitality can be taken internally as a dietary supplement.

All these bottled beauties help you to feel happy, collected and balanced. Simply having your hormones in harmony can make a HUGE difference in desire.

What if you suspect your hormones are off but you don't know which ones you need most. When in doubt, most women are too low in progesterone. Progessence Plus is a good place to start. You could also ask your Dr. to order blood work and test your hormone levels. At the back of this book, I have included frequently asked questions. The last page gives information on finding quality labs.

What about if you've had a hormone related disease? What if you are on birth control? How about if you are pregnant or nursing? All these questions are addressed by the Dr. himself in his frequently asked questions document which I have attached at the back.

Learning to use these oils has helped me to be more even keeled and resilient. I use a drop or two on my forearms as needed, then I go about my day. It helps put my estrogen and progesterone back into harmony similar to how I was before kids. Not only do they bring back sexual desire, they can improve general happiness and serenity as well. So many of my BFFs reported "being nicer to my kids" as a benefit. (I'm not kidding!) Balance is happiness inside the bedroom and out. Balance is strength and these bottles are the scorpion pose of balancing oils.

Notes

_____

_____

_____

_____

_____

_____

_____

Ylang Ylang™

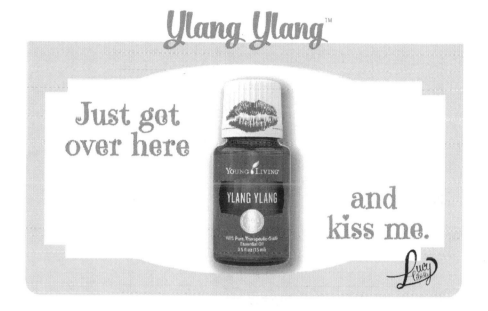

Just got over here and kiss me.

Ylang Ylang! *Ahhhhh!* Sweet delectable Ylang Ylang. I hope you have some. I hope so because that stuff is amazing. Its power as an aphrodisiac, has been long known. In Indonesia, the petals of the Ylang Ylang flowers are scattered over the bed of newlywed couples on their wedding night.

Ylang Ylang is one of the ingredients in both Joy and Sensation oil blends, and it is especially wonderful in my opinion because it increases libido in women and men tend to respond to the scent on their women as well.

Ylang Ylang is a flower that grows in Equador. The petals are picked early in the morning to maximize oil yield. The oil increases feeling of happiness, adoration, and it calms the mind and can even lower blood pressure just a tad to help you feel zen.

Ylang Ylang is known to harmonize and balance male-female energies. It increases libido in both men and women by increasing sexual energy. It can be used in the diffuser, and it is simply magical on the inner thighs.

Ylang Ylang is generally regarded as safe for consumption (GRAS = ingestible), however this oil smells so amazing that I would never put it in a capsule. This baby works best by building euphoria in the air, or by seducing him through having him inhale it from your thighs. It calls: "Just get over here and kiss me".

Notes

magic on the inner thighs

Cypress™

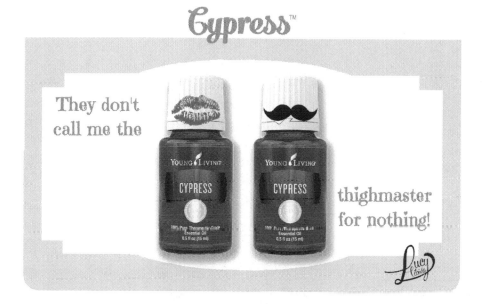

They don't call me the ... thighmaster for nothing!

Lucy

Cypress... *Yippee!!* We are back to Cypress again! I do believe I already ranted and raved about how awesome it is to tone down veins and any lumpity-lumps on your hiney. Time to talk about my *favorite* use of this lovely conifer. I call Cypress the "Thigh-master". It is my favorite oil to use in thigh blends for the bedroom. It can be used for men and women, but I have included it here because it is simply a MUST-HAVE to help the ladies get swollen in the flood gates.

You can mix Cypress with any other oil that you love. Cypress and Orange, Cypress and Ylang Ylang and Cypress and Clary Sage. You get the idea.

The reason I love Cypress so much for use between the sheets is because Cypress stimulates blood flow and circulation in the body. There is science behind it, but I like to think of it as a magical power that sucks all heat and blood from my legs upwards and inwards. Oh. My. Yes... Blood flow is kinda a big deal when you are talking squirming beneath the covers. If you need help getting engorged, Cypress is your friend. If you want him standing at attention like a saluting navy seal, then guess what?! That's going to depend a LOT on blood flow too. And likewise, super DUPER O-My-WOW explosions for her depend a lot on blood flow as well.

See the pattern? Cypress = blood flow and blood flow = magic. Apply it on your inner thighs. Apply it on his inner thighs. Mix it with your other favorites. But DON'T forget the Cypress. For the love of Lucy's favorite... Don't forget the Cypress.

Notes

If too strong cut Ylang Ylang or Joy w/ orange

Cypress increases blood flow

Clary Sage™

A girl's... best friend

Yay! Next we are going to talk about a girl's best Friend; Clary Sage.

Clary Sage is a lady's oil that has been used since once-upon-a-time for hormonal issues. It is your friend during PMS; while your Aunt Redina-Flow stops into town and for the hormonal drop after she leaves. Clary Sage is one of the main oils to help with PMS in our beloved Dragon Time, and to balance hormones in blends like Sclaressence and Lady Sclareol.

Right around that red time of the month, estrogen levels drop quickly and drastically. This is part of the reason why you may feel the need to break down crying when your cycliner doesn't go on straight. Everything is tragic when your estrogen levels are low.

But doesn't estrogen increase the risk of really scary tumors? Yes, and no. Women who naturally have higher levels of estrogen don't tend to take synthetic estrogen. Women who take synthetic estrogen hormonal therapy have higher rates of diseases. We talked about this a bit already with Progessence Plus, but it's good to recap. Studies have shown that SYNTHETIC estrogen (and progesterone) are linked to high disease rates as a side effect. And using plant compounds (such as P4 yam progesterone in Progressence Plus or phytoestrogens in Clary Sage) do not increase the risk of these scary side effects. In fact they have been shown to lower your risk in some studies.

OK- so where does this all tie in with Libido???? This is REALLY cool. You see, a woman naturally feels more "in the mood" when her estrogen levels are higher. This is because our estrogen levels are highest when we are ovulating. We are designed to feel more in the mood when we are fertile. It's how we were made.

As we age, our estrogen levels drop. One sign of low estrogen is "dryness" down there. Applying Clary Sage to the inner thighs or below the navel helps to increase natural lubrication. I can TOTALLY attest to that. Talk about the difference between a dry turkey and a juicy one. Want a really easy way to remember? Not to freak you out..., but you know that time you went to the bathroom and your TP was totally all slimy, opaque and creamy..... Yeah. *High estrogen day*. Now you will think of me every time it happens.

Using a drop of Clary Sage daily can increase your natural levels of estrogen that will help you feel more frisky, more lubricated, and more willing. You can apply on your forearms, wrists, Vitaflex points for the reproductive system, on the back of the neck or below the navel.

You can also diffuse Clary Sage. It's a middle note-which means it's not super floral or super earthy. It mixes well with bright top notes like Orange, or with floral blends like Ylang Ylang or Joy.

Clary Sage is also generally regarded as safe for internal consumption. If you choose to use Clary Sage internally, start with 1-2 drops in a capsule filled with Olive Oil. Note; this may make you more fertile.

So, to all the Lucy wannabes; If you want to be juicy, naturally lubed and frisky, start adding a drop of Clary Sage to your daily routine. You may find that you are a little more frisky and a lot more prepped downstairs for Mr. Libido.

Notes

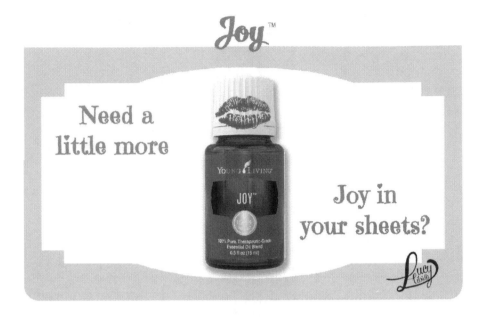

Joy. Joy makes me so joyful that I wrote a poem. Ahem.

Lucy's Ode to Joy

Oh Joy, how I love thee,
With your lovely floral scent that
replaced my paraben perfume.
Joy; who balances my crazy hormones,
Promotes feelings of self-worth,
And makes me irresistible to Mr. LiBido.

Okay. So it doesn't rhyme. I can't be good at everything. But, I could literally go on and on and ON about how much I love Joy. When I first got Joy it was in the Everyday Oils kit. I thought it would be one I wouldn't use much, but boy-oh-joy-oh-boy was I wrong! I love the way it smells and more importantly, how it makes me feel.

I use it over my heart during the day to balance out my crazy and to bring me a calm happy feeling. And my Mr. not only loves the attitude adjustment it gives, but he also can't seem to keep his hands off me. Yes, I bathe in Joy now.

Did you know that Joy was originally named "Love"? The oils in joy stimulate the brain and senses for love and affection. Diffusing Joy is a good way to invite the mood. If you don't love the aroma of Joy, try blending it with some Lemon to make it brighter or blend it with Clary Sage to make it less floral and earthier. This oil can be used aromatically or topically to raise frequency and to increase feelings of love.

And at Night? Oh at night… Take a couple of drops of Joy in a couple of drops of carrier (I personally love Sensation Massage Oil for this) and rub it on your inner thighs. Get all the way up in your leg crease, and on your lower abdomen. If your Mr. loves the floral scent - put a drop between your cleavage. Trust me. The perfect blend of oils like Ylang Ylang, Geranium, Jasmine and Rose really get you in the moooooooood. And when you are in the mood - it's always more juicy and delicious. I like to do this straight out of the shower right before getting into bed.

With Joy to help me, I have been able to get to the big "jOy" faster. So if you don't have it already - put it on your must-have list. If you have it already (lucky lucky), pull it out tonight. Your "Ode to Joy song will probably sound better than mine. Something more like:" Oh…… Ohhhhhhhhhhhhhh……

OHHHHHH………JOOOOOOOOYYYY!!!!!

topically on the ♡ w/ orange, clary sage & orange

Sensation™

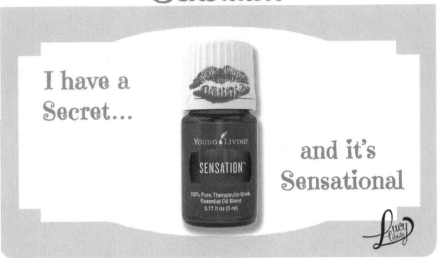

I have a Secret...

and it's Sensational

I've got a *secret.* And it's sensational. And it's like something else we're talking about here.... it also starts with the letter S.

That little secret is Sensation.

Sensation is an alluring blend that is a mix of Ylang Ylang, Rosewood and Jasmine. It smells like Joy, but a little bit softer because it lacks the Geranium that gives Joy its strong floral scent. Not a lot of people know about Sensation..... but it's named that for a reason. It is simply *Sensational.*

It really gets me purrrrring. Often, I find myself feeling over scheduled and stressed to the point that it makes me not want to be touched. Boo. When I am in this state, Sensation can help pull me out and help release my blocks to being intimate and loved. I find the scent to be uplifting and opening.

Sensation can be used aromatically to set the tone. The soft floral aroma is uplifting and arousing without being overbearing. When Mr. Libido smells our room full of Sensation, he knows what's in store for the two of us.

My favorite way to use Sensation is on the inner thighs. You can use it on the edge of your ears, the back of the neck, and in your cleavage crease too. The moment I apply a couple of drops of Sensation to these areas, I start to have feelings of ANTICIPATION. My body starts tingling and I begin to crave what's next.

I love it mixed with orange, or cypress, or even all by itself. Sensation is so mild that it can even be used on more sensitive areas with very little dilution. Have your Mr. Libido rub a drop of coconut oil and a couple drops of Sensation all over your C-singing love button and Oh, WOW! You will not be complaining. You'll be singing. "Lucy was Right this is O O O soooooo Sensational!!!!

Notes

_____

_____

_____

_____

_____

_____

_____

_____

Valor™

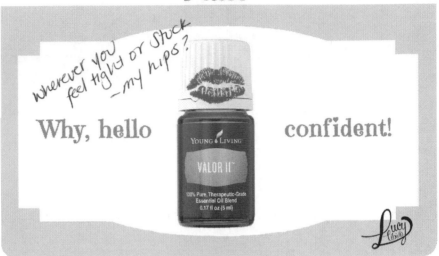

wherever you feel tight or stuck — my hips?

Why, hello confident!

If you are yet to *discover* Valor, you don't know what you are missing. There's a reason it's the number one sought after oil for emotional health. Every girlfriend should have a bottle of Valor on hand. Valor is fabulous for loosing emotional blocks. Valor contains oils that stimulate the limbic area of the brain and helps you to relax and promote feelings of confidence and courage. This is the perfect oil to use throughout the day to keep stress levels down in general. In the bedroom, it smells amazing when diffused. You can wear Valor over your heart, or on the wrists or brainstem on the back of the neck.

Valor helps me to ease feeling of anxiousness and worry. If Valor could talk, she would say "Don't worry, It's going to be OK". And oddly enough, even though Valor can't talk, she says this to your mind when you put it on your body. And when she reassures you, you believe her.

Valor is the perfect "preparation oil". Wear it while you are shaving your legs, making an inner thigh roller bottle or when you are picking out something smashing to wear. Valor makes you confident about whatever is imminent. So, you can feel self-assured during the day at the office, and fearless at night in the bedroom.

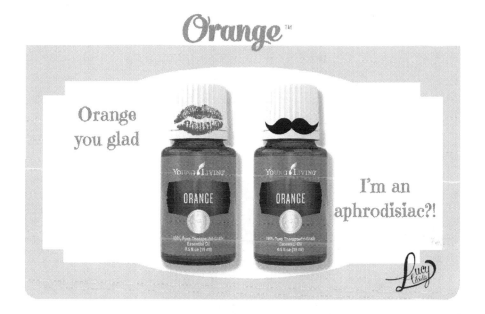

Orange. Orange is like a drop of *happiness* in a bottle. It's one of the sweetest and most brightly amber saturated oils in the rainbow. Orange is a "bright" oil. Orange welcomes light and happiness. It is carefree and secure. Orange brightens the mood, lifts the spirit, energizes the mind and creates feelings of bliss. Think of summer childhood days playing in the water or eating bright popsicles out in the sun.

For the adult, Orange helps to let go of stress and enjoy being in the moment. This oil opens the sacral chakra near the pelvic area. This chakra is associated with pleasure, creativity, and sensuality. Orange is an aphrodisiac oil that helps you to let go of your grown-up problems and embrace sexuality and fun. Orange is AWESOME for frigidity. It can help you relax if you have low libido due to a bit of anxiety. It is fantastic when mixed with a floral like Ylang Ylang or an equalizer like Cypress or Clary Sage.

It can be used in the diffuser, to help you chill, or on the inner thighs to unwind and let go.

Orange also earns a rockstar status for the man. In order for a man's joystick to perform like the 1984 Nintendo champion, he's got to have a plethora of hormones surging through his body in just the right order and at just the right time. It's kinda like having the secret code to unlock ultimate invincibility for hormonal success. Ask him if he remembers the ultimate code: Up-Down-Up-Down-Left-Right-Left-Right-B-A-B-A-Select-START. KABOOM!

Components of a man's secret joystick code are L-arginine, Testosterone, and Glutathione. L-arginine is an amino acid that improves Nitric Oxide in the body. Nitric Oxide improves vascular dilatation of the joystick. L-arginine can be found in natural supplements like MultiGreens. Glutathione is an antioxidant that is concentrated in the liver. 8 topical drops of Orange or Lime oil can increase his own internal glutathione levels dramatically. This is because they contain high levels of citrol and d-limonene which stimulate glutathione production in the body. So, add some Orange or Lime oil to his daily routine. Aside from smelling like a carefree summer popsicle, it will support his Big Stick as well.

Notes

_____

_____

_____

_____

Libido it Up. Oils for Him

Idaho Blue Spruce™

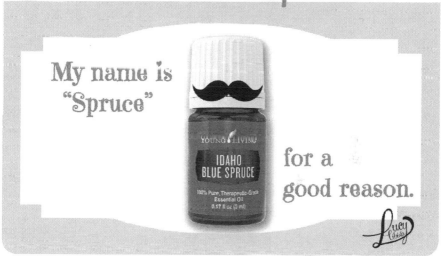

My name is "Spruce" for a good reason.

Lucy LiBido

All right, now we get to chat more about oils for the men. While many of these oils can be used on both genders (Orange, Cypress, Mister for example), some are especially suited to just him. We're going to start with one of my favorite oils for HIM. And by that, I mean an oil that your main man can wear to make sex more awesome for you. Because let's face it... when intimacy is better for you, it happens more often for HIM. That's something that Mr. LiBido wants to pass along to all the men out there!

Mr. LiBido has an oil that he really likes. It's called Idaho Blue Spruce. And it really does "SPRUCE" him up in a very good way. It helps him stay firmer longer so I can enjoy myself longer as well. It's nature's version of that little blue hexagon, if you will. This sprucing oil is like a military call to STAND at ATTENTION! It can be used with coconut oil as a lubricant and has a nice cooling effect for me too. It is just one oil of many that we like to use, to make intimacy last longer.

Dr. Dan Purser shared that 8 drops a day of Idaho Blue Spruce in a capsule showed a 30% increase in testosterone in 2 weeks. Some report higher levels in the same time frame, and I know of many who keep their levels high with only 5 drops. Some of my friends have even reported that with regular ingestion, their man has seen actual lengthening in their little soldier. The things I talk about with my girlfriends!

Here's the nice thing about it... your man isn't left with any "unmanageable salutes", as my dear husband would say. It wears off naturally soon after intercourse. BUT it keeps things going longer and helps with firmness. Yes, I could tell a difference. I'm not promising actual numbers.... and NO, I will not include a before and after picture with a ruler. But for the sake of learning, let's just say that the first time we used this oil, I instantly saw and FELT a difference. As for you, it's fine for a little to rub off you internally. It's warming and exotic. It's a must-have oil in the bedroom!

Idaho Blue Spruce can be used aromatically, topically and internally. I do like how this one smells in the air. If you want to use it in a massage oil for both of you, it can be blended with one of the more feminine oils like Ylang Ylang.

You can (and when I say "you can" I mean "you should") use Idaho Blue Spruce in a warm-up session. This is where I remind you again to dilute and apply to the forearm first. After your forearm gives the go ahead, then go ahead and apply to his inner thighs and the lower shaft of his soldier. I don't recommend applying over the eye of the one-eyed-snake. Oils don't go in eyes. Even snake eyes.

If your man just needs a little boost, it's amazing what a little "wake-up call" capsule can do for him. Have him take a capsule with 3-5 drops Idaho Blue Spruce 20 minutes before go-time.

Then manually massage some more (diluted) around his lower shaft and love stones for an extra sturdy soldier. If your man needs help in the firmness department, has low libido, or needs some assistance with longevity or standing at attention, then daily internal use would yield a better result than occasional usage in the bedroom. He can take 3-8 drops in a capsule with olive oil as a supplement for men's health. Who knew a conifer could be SOOO Spruce-tastic?!

Notes

Slight tingle

5 drops / day internally increases testosterone

Goldenrod™

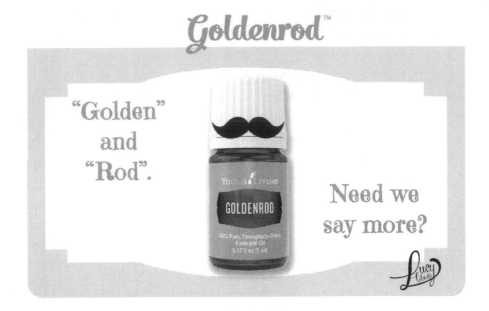

"Golden" and "Rod".

Need we say more?

Goldenrod! Ahhhhhhh Goldenrod. *Tee hee hee.* I can hardly say the name without snickering. Let me tell you a story. Once upon a time, there was a plant named "Goldenrod." The essential oil from the flowering top of the plant was found to improve circulation and aid the urinary tract. According to the University of Montreal in Canada, it was also found to help with deflated hoses and firmness of.... well, you know... that male body part we've come to refer to around here as, "the Soldier." I told my friends about this lovely, blessed oil and its USEFUL advantages, and they gave it a try. My friends reported back an increase in firmness using goldenrod topically as well as internally.

We've come to love Goldenrod so much that we don't call it "Goldenrod" anymore. We call it Golden ROD. Cuz, truly Golden + Rod..... that's what it does. This is very good news for those who want a little more GOLD in their ROD.

Goldenrod is a seasonal oil that is distilled in the fall. I highly recommend stocking up in the fall to have plenty to last you through the spring. It's a sad day when you tip your goldenrod bottle upside down and it's empty in March. All the Valentine

Day lovers snatched it up in February and there are months to wait until it blooms again.

You can use Goldenrod topically in a soldier and love stone massage or as an inner thigh love potion.

You can also choose to take up to 3 drops in a capsule. Goldenrod oil has long been known to be edible ever since the Boston Tea Party era, when English tea was dumped in the harbor and the colonists drank Goldenrod tea instead. My Mr. Libido has used it in a perky pill with much success. A little goes a long way. Enjoy your golden "rod" ladies!

Notes

_____

_____

_____

_____

_____

_____

_____

_____

Nutmeg™

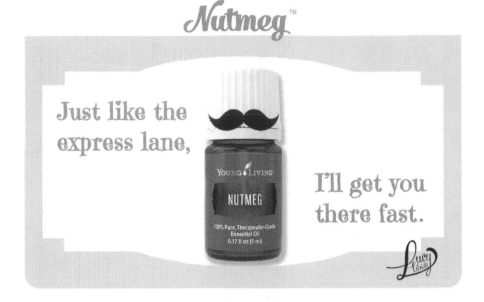

Just like the express lane,

I'll get you there fast.

Oohhhhhh *Ok.* Nutmeg is another blood pumping must-have for your Mister. Technically, it can be used on the ladies too, but we've seen the best results using it for the guys. You ready for some fun facts?

Nutmeg essential oil is extracted by steam distillation from seed or husk of the Myristica fragrans plant. It is a stimulant. Applied over the belly or taken internally (only Young Living Vitality of course). Nutmeg improves digestion by stimulating the stomach. It has long been known to help with issues like flatulence, and indigestion and constipation.

Now, before you say "Ew that's not what I'm here for Lucy", Nutmeg is also an aphrodisiac oil. Nutmeg's stimulating property stimulates energy, both physical and sexual energy. Some people report feeling "wired" after diffusing or ingesting Nutmeg. And it can be comparable to a caffeine kick depending on your body's chemistry.

Nutmeg is an aphrodisiac because emotionally, it stimulates energy and physicality, because it increases circulation and acts as a vasodilator. Vaso=blood vessels and dilator=makes bigger. Put two and two together. I think you can do the math.

Nutmeg is such an effective tool for dilating blood vessels and increasing circulation that it is the first natural recommendation for Raynauds - a condition where the blood vessels constrict.

Nutmeg is SO stimulating, that it can have negative effects when used in large amounts, like, heart racing, or palpitations, or hallucinations. So, don't go crazy. No drinking a whole bottle in hopes to transform into Captain America okay?

Nutmeg can be diffused, taken internally, or applied topically. It's a little more sensitizing on the skin than Goldenrod or Idaho Blue Spruce; so be sure to DILUTE this one and start on the inner thighs and work "up" from there only IF needed. Usually, I keep this one on the inner thighs. Internally, I recommend starting with 1-2 vitality drops diluted with olive oil in a capsule.

If energy in the bedroom is what you're after - try this fun little recipe. This special blend is called "Lucy's Perky Pill" and it is the result of fun-time trial and error in our research group. After you have ensured that your arm doesn't have any sensitivity to these oils, make the perky capsule.

It's 5 drops Idaho Blue Spruce, 3 drops Goldenrod, and 3 drops Nutmeg in a capsule with 10 drops Olive Oils. Have him take 10-30 minutes before go time.

Tell your Mr. not to double the recipes just because he has bulging muscles like Thor. Even Thor should start with the classic recipe. I should know. We're tight.

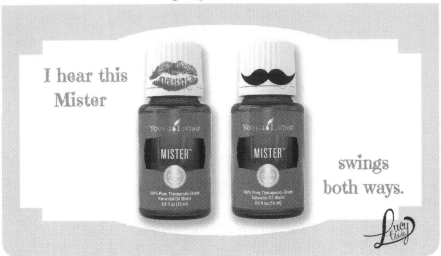

Next, we will be discussing a special oil blend for the hubsters called Mister. This blend was originally formulated to balance male energy and support healthy prostate function. Ironically, some women found that it ALSO helped them with hot flashes and mood swings.

Remember when we were talking earlier that hot flashes, PMS, irritability and night sweats are often a sign of low progesterone or low estrogen?

Well, occasionally they can be a sign of hormonal imbalance where your estrogen is too high and testosterone too low. I know, it sounds crazy! Not enough testosterone. But we contain them all. And for women who are estrogen dominant, adding estrogen to their lives (even if it's natural) doesn't make them more balanced obviously.

Women who tend to feel more balanced using Mister fall in the category of being estrogen dominant, and they tend to be older than 30. But, that's not a hard fast rule.

Mister is a blend that is designed to balance male hormones, support prostate health and help it to function properly. Mister contains an oil called Blue Yarrow. That same Blue Yarrow is also in our beloved Dragon Time blend. So, it can help balance the glandular system in both men and women.

Dragon time tends to help women ages puberty through 30 and Mister tends to work well for women 30+. Again, this is a general guideline, and either age group could use either oil.

As for men, Mister helps the prostate function optimally therefore it can be a big part of his libido and performance. You can apply Mister to his ankles and the front and back pubic bones. Apply daily for optimal prostate performance. It smells quite nice actually, and it's really soothing in a bath, or worn as a cologne.

The ingredients of Mister are: Yarrow - a prostate decongestant and hormone balancer, Sage - strengthens vital centers, Myrtle - helps normalize hormonal imbalances of the thyroid and sex glands, Fennel - has hormone-like activity, Lavender - is relaxing and grounding, and Peppermint - strengthens the liver and glandular function. All good things to get the man back on track.

As a total tangent and side note - I've been to the Young Living farm and I have watched them distill Blue Yarrow. This is an oil that is hard to find. It is absolutely fascinating. The flowers are a pale yellow - but the oil comes out a bright blue. During the distillation process, the plant material releases chamazulene which gives the oil its vivid blue color. And that's what gives the light blue tint to your Dragon Time and Mister blend.

If your husband's libido gas tank is running low, this is definitely one to look into to perk things up again. Or even possibly yours. Mister isn't picky; this blend swings both ways.

Hong Kuai™

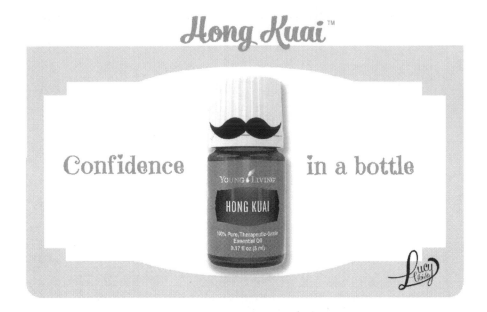

Confidence in a bottle

Remember when we talked about how it's more important to feel confident than it is to look like a Barbie Doll? Well, Hong Kuai is often called "confidence in a bottle". With the highest sesquiterpene content of all aphrodisiac oils, Hong Kuai is like inhaling liquid confidence.

Hong Kuai is distilled from trees that grow on the steep rainforest mountaintops of Taiwan. I imagine that whoever can get up there to retrieve these trees must have already had some given to them from their Tarzan ancestors. Who else would have such confidence and courage to ascend to the tops of the earth for such a priceless oil? They probably have developed grappling muscles from climbing, smell of deep woody pheromones and can captivate their ladies like Mr. Libido. But, I digress.

Hong Kuai trees typically live 1,000-2,000 years. Each year they produce a new tree ring having its own deposit of that year's essential oil. It's as if it proposes a new ring each and every year to the Tarzans who are collecting confidence for their beloved Janes. The masculine woody aroma is perfect worn daily as cologne, or can be mixed with Idaho Blue Spruce for the ultimate blend of mental and physical fortitude.

Notes

liquid confidence

Shutran™

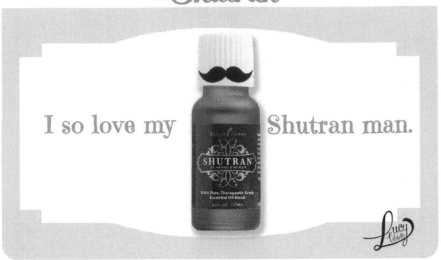

I so love my Shutran man.

ALL RIGHT. I saved the *BEST* for the last. At least, that's how I feel. SHUTRAN!

Shutran is one of the newer blends and was released to an intrigued crowd in Salt Lake City. Because of the nature of announcing things publicly - it was referred to as "Cologne". The online description vaguely states, "Just a few drops throughout the day will help with an impossible workday or the pursuits of a special evening." At first, I was like - who's gonna spend that much on cologne????

But Oh! MY OH MY! Shutran is more than a cologne. Shutran is the first and ONLY oil created specifically to help catch a lady's attention. Remember when you learned about the science of essential oils (nod your head yes); remember that it's not the scent that is effective - but the chemical constituents inside the oil. Shutran is formulated for a man to wear - to help turn on the lady. It's like a bottle of sweet smelling pheromones wafting into the hidden parts of your brain, stimulating your naughtiest imagination. Once you realize what Shutran does... Oh, THEN it becomes worth every penny.

Shutran is good for the guy AND the girl! I personally love the scent. MMMMMmmmmmmmm. When Mr. LiBido puts on a couple drops on his neck like cologne, I MELT!! Then I can't keep my hands off him. Ahh, I love it! It's perfectly blended with man boosting oils like Hinoki tree oil, but doesn't smell too "woodsy". It smells, really.... really... attractive.

Now, what does Shutran do for the man?? Let's just say that it's loaded with Idaho Blue Spruce, which we all know is like a hexagon of happiness. It makes sense that Idaho Blue Spruce is a key ingredient in Shutran. Apply a drop to the shaft. Rub it in.... Oh girls... You will love your Shutran Man!

He can use Shutran topically on the forearms, on the shaft, or the inner thighs. He can wear it daily (like a cologne) to boost testosterone and confidence. It can also be used topically on the woman on the forearms, or on the inner thighs. Some ladies find that it really gets them going too. Women should use it right beforehand as opposed to daily. It also can be diffused to build the mood - seriously this one smells AMAZING.

K, in our little group of Lucy ladies... we have a slogan. We say it all the time. We randomly drop it to each other as messages. We say it under our breath as we walk past. We can't say it enough. Our mantra... "I love my Shutran Man!"

Don't forget the Love Button

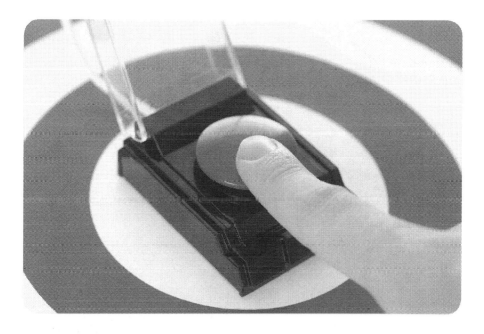

Hello, hello, hello! I saved some of the best topics and stories for the end. After I taught a libido oils class to 10,000 of my closest BFFs, I started to get a lot of messages. Chapter 9 is based off of listening to numerous women who want help finishing their nights in awe and wonder.

I have learned that so many women struggle to climax. It does not come with the same ease as it does in their manly other half. Well, I have a secret.... Men and women work differently in the bedroom. Surprise!!

We're going to jump out of the sheets and into our biology books for just a moment here. Time for my cat-eye reading glasses.

When a young fetus is developing, it has unisex genitalia with nerve endings that are exactly the same for boys and girls. This ambiguous genitalia looks like a little bud or bump with a small opening underneath. At this time, hormones and androgens determine whether this sweet little kidney bean will become a Larry or a Lacey. If the genital tube is exposed to testosterone, then the little opening will fuse, grow testes and the little bud will elongate outward becoming our stalwart soldier for Larry. If there is a lack of testosterone, then the small opening will enlarge inward towards a uterus and the little bump will remain as the female clitoris. Or, the love button, as I like to call it.

The majority of pleasurable nerve endings for both females and males stem from this same little bump. These nerve endings are what are responsible creating the waves of pleasure and the rush of oxytocin that flood our bodies during climax.

So why is this important? Well, many, MANY women struggle with climax. For men it is simple; their nerve endings are at the tips of their soldier and it's PRETTY impossible not to stimulate them when storming the beach. For women, it's a little more complicated. Numerous studies have shown that about 80% of women are unable to climax with intercourse alone. Only 20% of women receive adequate stimulation with penetration in order to consistently climax without manual stimulation. And while there are nerve endings inside us which do make love making enjoyable, the majority of those that finish the deed are outside the cave. So, in a group of 10,000, that means about 8,000 needs some type of love button massage to finish the night totally and feel totally and completely satisfied.

Don't you feel better that you aren't alone? I sure did!

It has nothing to do with how tall or wide his soldier salutes nor does it have anything to do will how sexy or fantastic you are as a woman. Our love buttons are equal to his soldier in terms of what they do. They need friction to make them happy. And only a few of us happen to get enough love button massage movement through penetration.

Just knowing this will make your whole world a lot brighter. You are perfectly normal if you don't start wailing at the drop of your bra and start singing the Good Ship Lollipop after 3 thrusts in. You (and he) have got to know how to turn on the love button.

Now, I'm not going to provide a step-by-step directions, nor give you advice on techniques or positions (there are already plenty of books on that), but I'll give you some pointers on maximizing your love button exposure.

First – a woman's love button swells with blood JUST like when your man's Soldier stands at attention. When it swells, the tissue presses outward and forward so that the most sensitive parts are exposed and are more likely to be stimulated. Foreplay is necessary for a woman to swell. This includes hugs, kisses, cuddles, touching, stroking and massage. These things are vital. If your Mr. is going spelunking before warming you up and rubbing you down, you aren't going to get the same pull and play if you were engorged and excited. I've had people tell me that their Mr. skips this because it gets him soooooo worked up that he shoots and misses the basket before the game has even begun. If this is the case, I tell them that his turn is over and she still gets to play. Put a condom on that puppy to slow him down. She comes first.

Second, change it up and position yourselves so that the love button is either being stimulated by rubbing against his body, or in such a way that he (or you) can simultaneously massage it at the same time. There are also more nerve endings at the front wall of your indoor waterslide (known as the G spot). You can locate it by inserting a finger and making a "come here" motion towards the belly button. Some women really enjoy this area being stimulated with either a finger or with his saluting joystick. These are the two most important places to be hitting to create the most pleasure. So, unless your man has an unusually upward curving joystick, and some random but conveniently placed mole above his Soldier... well, then you're not going to be hitting your G-spot or love button in the missionary position...

Thirdly, strengthen the pelvic floor muscles that contract during the big O. Especially after childbirth, these pelvic muscles tend to get stretched out and weak. But just like any muscle, they will increase in strength with regular exercise. Kegel exercises involve using the muscles that you would use if you were in the bathroom, and stopped the flow of urine. Tighten, Hold, Release and Repeat. That's it. Now, do it 50 times every day. Pick a time you'll always remember…. like after you go to the bathroom, while you're brushing your teeth, while you're in the shower etc. You can even get a little kinky and do them on your lunch break while you are chatting with your co-workers. They'll think you are thinking about your salad, when in reality you'll be kegeling away for a better romp in the hay all while looking them straight in the face. Muhahahaha. I've done it.

Then when you come home from your lunch, focus on holding these muscles while you are with Mr. Libido. Contracting these muscles tightens the pelvic floor around the pudendel nerve - which is deeply embedded into the pelvic floor, and sends messages of pleasure from the nerves in the love button to the brain. You want to hug that nerve. It makes you happy. It also makes Mr. Libido happy because squeezing and strengthening those muscles creates a firmer grip for him.

Last but not least. SO important. Use a love button massage oil. If you haven't yet…. then your whole world is about to change. You can use it to get you warmed up, to keep things exciting while you enjoy each other, or simply to just make you explode.

OH MY! IT'S GETTING A LITTLE HOT IN HERE. I need to cross my legs. Ohhhhhh…

And because I'm recommending a love button massage oil, I'm going to share my favorites in our recipe section. Lucky you.

Other Hotshots for the Bedroom

Shutran Shave Cream™   Mirah Shave Oil™

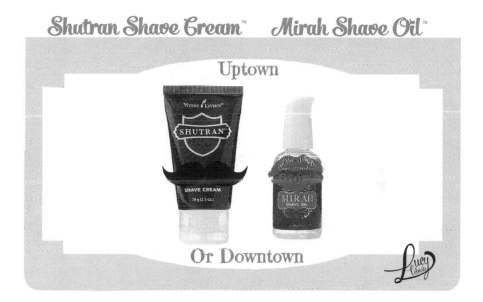

Uptown

Or Downtown

I'm not the one to tell people what to wear, or how to style their hair, but if you've appreciated my guidance this far, then this little tip may be of service to you.

We've already touched on why physical and mental preparation gets us ready emotionally, how Shutran makes a lady melt, and how important it is to provide a rub-a-dub party for the love button.

When you go to the hairdresser, she may give you stylist tips - like your face shape will look better with layers or your hair texture is suited better to a long or short cut. We're going to talk a leeeeetle bit about your downtown stylist.

There is no right or wrong way to wear your locks, however, if you fall into the category of 75-80% of women who do not climax with penetration alone, you (and HE) would probably benefit from a downtown pixie cut over braids.

Why's this? Well remember how the love button needs lots of time and attention? The smoother and slicker it is, the better. Keeping her South Pole kissers smooth and free of excess fibers creates a smoother uninterrupted escapade.

And Mr. Libido? If a pixie cut suits her well, then a military buzz may be for him. Keeping any areas above his solider soft as buttah will enhance her experience allowing her happy places to slide against wet tile rather than shag carpet.

Getting ready and shaving in the shower is a physical and mental preparation for me. Being trim and prepared makes me excited all day and mentally get me ready. He has taken note as well, learning from experience that I am happier when he is smooth enough in all the right places. So imagine my excitement when Shutran shave gel made its appearance alongside Mirah Shave Oil. It's as if they were made for me.

Aphrodisiac oils can be blended with anything that you love. One of my favorite aromas is Lemon Myrtle, so I tend to add that to my diffuser blends. Here are a few other oils I always have on hand to mix into my love potions.

Sandalwood – Grounding and balancing, this sensual woody aroma stimulates the pineal gland and is spiritually enlightening.

Black Pepper – Spicy and warm, this oil is a good addition to stimulating lubes. It stimulates and warms on contact. A little goes a long way. Dilute.

Peppermint – Minty and cool, this oil give a crisp and tingling sensation to love lubes. Remember that peppermint is very strong and must be heavily diluted or it can burn mucous membranes.

Tea Tree / Melaleuca Alternifolia – Tea Tree oil gives a minty-hot sensation to love lubes. If you are prone to yeast infections,

I would highly recommend adding Tea Tree oil to all your homemade (or store bought) lubes because it inhibits the growth of yeast. This one is also too strong to use neat; dilute in a lube.

Clove or Thieves – Clove or Thieve are the ideal oils to have on hand for oral pleasure. Lightly dilute them and apply to the roof of the mouth using your thumb. They will numb the back of the throat and help with gag reflex. It can also be mixed with peppermint for this purpose, to make a "cinnamint" oral blend. Do not apply directly to genitals.

Jasmine – Jasmine is a floral oil that invokes feelings of femininity and love. It's one of the oils in Joy and it smells beautiful as a perfume. The top note blends well with Clary Sage, Cypress, or Sandalwood.

Grapefruit – I use this in edible body butters because dang; it just tastes good.

Lime – I also use this in edible concoctions because it's got a nice flavor, and it is high in D-Limonene which improves glutathione levels. Yum and yay.

Light the Fire - This blend will really light your fire. It's spicy and sweet and it fiery in love lubes. Dilute and be careful!

Real Women; Real Stories

Hi Lucy!

Just wanted to let you know some ways your class helped!

I'm in my mid-fifties; Progessence Plus has been wonderful to help libido, dryness, and to help me "get there" faster and of course that makes my hubby feel very successful!

Idaho Blue Spruce, Shutran, and Mister are three of his favorite oils, applied to wrists, neck, and groin beforehand and in a lube right on his "soldier" during... He hasn't needed that little pill that he previously used.

The various YLEO's including Idaho Blue Spruce, Goldenrod, Sensation in a coconut oil carrier were great for both of us. Still tweaking the combinations to see what we like best. I'm excited to keep learning! Thanks!

I.L

Me, I swear by Progessence Plus. I had chemical induced menopause. Using this oil in opinion has reversed it. I had a life threatening disease that required treatment that damaged my immune system. The side effect of this treatment was stopping my periods and my Dr. confirmed that it induced early menopause at only 41. I started using Progessence Plus regularly; my hot flashes were no more. The unexplained aches and pains were less, the tingling "electric" type feelings in my arms were gone, and my periods came back! I have never been so excited to have my period back. Using Progessence Plus has reversed the menopausal symptoms and brought me back to normal.

Jennifer M.

So, just reading through all the descriptions of all the oils when I first got started, I read about Mister, and thought it would be a good oil to try on my boyfriend. "Promotes inner-body balance that soothes stress," sounded perfect for my man! I really didn't know where to apply it, so I diluted it with a carrier oil and applied it to his belly/liver area with my bare hands. This was our nightly routine for about a week, when I realized I was in the mood ALL THE TIME!!! SO – I read up and yes! Some of the ingredients help enhance libido! Soooo to cut long story short, I think I benefited from the Mister more than him! I apply a drop to my inner ankles when I feel like being a little frisky.

Sarah S.

Joy!!! The first time I put this on my heart... was probably one of the best nights of our lives! I was brought to tears from the passion!

Bridget Bergstrom

Um, sensation?... You mean PANTY DROPPER AND IM 18 again... HORMONES?! Yes. Yes you are correct. Sensational. Thank you.

Julianne H.

Lucy, your class has been a Godsend to me and my husband. He struggles with E.D. that makes it difficult for him to be intimate. It has been a struggle on both of us. He started a popular medication for his problem, only to have major side effects with his heart. The stress it was causing on his heart wasn't safe, and we had to discontinue with despair thinking there was no solution.

I took your Lucy Libido class and learned about the testosterone increasing and performance encouraging oils. We started using Idaho Blue Spruce and IT HAS BROUGHT HIM BACK. He is so thankful and I am too. I am going to find you and hug you one day.

T.K.

I LOVE, LOVE, LOVE CLARY SAGE! Using it has completely corrected my hormonal imbalance. I use 2 drops in a dollop of coconut oil and rub across my lower back...my sides and sometimes my breasts...

Warning... it has caused me to have very vivid wildly sexual dreams of my husband of 22 years... our mornings are fabulous!!

Kimberly Priddy-Green

Can I share a secret? After having a baby, I started to feel a bit... broken. I wanted to love my husband, I wanted to be intimate. All the *want* was up in my head and there was a big disconnect between my brain and my *ahem* lady garden. No matter how good things felt, they just weren't feeling good enough to finish satisfied. And that was frustrating for both of us. I was feeling like all hope was lost, until you clued me into the wonders of Cypress and Orange on the inner thighs.

Orange helped me get out of my own head and relax. Cypress improved circulation, for me, means I'm much more sensitive to touch which has benefited me tremendously! I'm less anxious and it helps me find my happy place!

Jessica K.

I have been using Clary Sage non-stop since the class, and I really think it has helped me with my emotions!!! I feel more normal if that makes sense.

Sherrie B.

I can only say that the Progessence Plus along with the Dragon Time has changed my cycle in mind-blowing ways. I definitely feel that extending to my mood, my attitudes, how approachable I am, things like that. I've also been having a lot of chiropractic work done in the sacral area to help reset the nerve that extend to the reproductive organs and that has almost been amazing; and I think it's a combination of all these modalities that has changed me for the better. I applied both oils morning and night and then the dragon time more often during my cycle. I ordered my husband the Mister for some of his issues, and then next month he's getting Shutran. I can tell a huge difference if I miss any of this hormone balancing oils; I'll find myself mid-morning really off & then it hits me "oh! I know what's up with me; I didn't put my oils on!" My regular midwife was super supportive of the use of these oils. When traditional midwives employed by large hospitals are referring patients out for oil consults for hormone balancing, it shows that these oils really work!

Kellie L.S. Tucker

Progessence Plus, is a game changer. I have experienced great benefits using this oil such as decreased mood swings, improved PMS (I no longer want to bite your head off one minute and cry the other) weight loss, increased libido shortened and lighter menstrual periods. Overall, it's a great oil for total hormone balance. I apply 2 drops on the back of neck, twice a day and everyone is happy!!!

Crystal Catron

OMG! After trying Idaho Blue Spruce once, my hubby is asking for this to be used on him regularly! I LOVE it! He doesn't have problems in this department, but this helps it more! I used a 5ml roller. Used 10 drops and rest fractionated coconut oil. I rolled the base of his shaft all around and about 1 inch upward. I use it as foreplay and his "soldier" will be VERY firm!

Laura B.

Ever since having my boys, I was no longer interested in sex. Someone suggested Progessence Plus to me. So I bought it, popped a roller top on it and applied to my forearms. Took me a couple weeks to notice anything. But once I did notice.... wow. It was like I was back to my pre kid sex drive. Now, I don't have to use it every day like in the beginning. I can use it once or twice a week and still be good.

Becky H.

I learned about Progessence Plus when using it for migraines... and yes, you hit the nail on the head with that one! Lol, it definitely helped. Side effect though is waaay increased libido so watch out! Haha!

Nicara N.

Ylang Ylang. Yes. I got a bottle six months ago. I'm six months pregnant. Lol.

A. K.

Oh my goodness! Used Sensation on my wrists earlier this afternoon, then again on upper thighs 20 min before, and whoa! This stuff is seriously amazing! It was so easy to "get in the mood" and early on the orgasms came in waves! I was soooo sensitive in the best way possible. This mama feels sexy and blessed.

J.A.

Clary Sage was amazing for me during labor, kept me going and balanced my mind when all I wanted to do was quit!

Kaitlyn Bartz

CYPRESS. This is the real deal ladies. I'm just saying....

Shawna Coker

I learned in the Lucy Libido class last year about Idaho Blue Spruce acting as a "little blue pill" of sorts. So, I asked my Mister if he wanted to give it a shot, so he did! He applied 2 drops of the Idaho Blue Spruce to his "soldier" and we went to town.

It totally delivered and he went a lot longer than her normally would and actually got TIRED! Haha. We continued to use the IBS for our sexy time, and it's helped him have more energy and stamina- and he lasts longer! WIN/WIN all around!

Sarah S.

I used to spend $110-$175 on cologne that smelled fantastic, but wore off in an hour and did not have any holistic benefits. Now, I only wear essential oils and Shutran is a daily favorite! I always get a bottle in my stocking from Santa.

Ryan Burris

I noticed I was much nicer...much calmer, and more like ME after a few days usage of Progessence Plus. I use it 2x daily ...rollerball top on and apply on neck and forearms.

Tasha Walters

Dear Lucy – I tried Sensation, Ylang Ylang and Orange like you suggested. Assignment complete! Lucy, hear me say YOU ARE A GENIUS!! We are losing sleep. My husband wanted to know what happened to me and I told him about Lucy Libido group. Let's just say he is a fan!

Crystal Catron

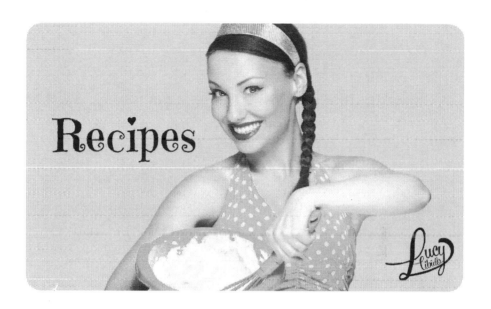

Recipes

Here they are! Lucy's favorite recipes. Theres something for everyone here. Diffuser recipes, Inner thigh blends, edible lubes, and even Mr. Libido's perky pill. Having fun between the sheets has never felt so natural!!

Mood Enhancing Diffuser Blends

Light some candles & choose your favorite diffuser blend.

Oooh La La

4 Drops Sensation

2 Drops Hong Kuai

2 Drops Lavender

Romantic Bliss

3 Drops Jasmine

2 Drops Orange

2 Drops Clary Sage

1 Drop Joy

Naughty and Nice

4 Drops Light the Fire

2 Drops Idaho Blue Spruce

2 Drops Orange

Yin and Yang

3 Drops Sandalwood

3 Drops Lavender

2 Drops Ylang Ylang

Here I Come

3 Drops Joy

3 Drops Lemon Myrtle

2 Drops Nutmeg

Confident

5 Drops Valor

3 Drops Hong Kuai

Natural Lubes for Him and Her

These chemical-free lubes are designed to keep you juicy and tender while you stuff the turkey.

Lucy's Love Lube

3 Tablespoons Sensation Massage Oils blended with

12 Drops Sensation
8 Drops Cypress
8 Drops Orange
4 Drops Peppermint

Whipped Mousse

1/4 Cup solid coconut
1/4 Cup refined shea butter
1 tsp Sweet almond oil
25 Drops Shutran
25 Drops Ylang Ylang
10 Drops Cypress
10 Drops Clary Sage

Whip the coconut and shea butter in a high speed mixer for 2 minutes.

Add sweet almond and essential oils, then use generously and often!

Sweet and Warm

3 Tablespoons solid coconut whipped with

10 Drops Tea Tree
10 Drops Ylang Ylang
10 Drops Lavender
5 Drops Clary Sage
3 Drops Black Pepper

Latex Friendly Vera Lube

Got latex? This recipe is oil-free for condom fun. It also feels SO good that you'll want to slather it up your hoo-ha regardless of needing a condom.

2 tsp Trader Joe's aloe vera
2 Teaspoons water
1/2 Teaspoons glycerin
1/2 Teaspoon Vitamin E

Blend and enjoy!

The Quickie
Sensation Massage Oil

Coconut oil and essential oils have not been studied for condom compatibility. Use at your own risk when relying on a condom.

Inner Thigh Potions

For him and for her, apply from the inner mid-thigh to the leg crease. Make ahead and store in a 5ml bottle. Keep it in the bedroom!!

Her

Sweet Thing
20 Drops Ylang Ylang
20 Drops Cypress
5 Drops Lavender
25 Drops Carrier

Sensational
25 Drops Sensation
10 Drops Cypress
5 Drops Jasmine
25 Drops Carrier

Juicy
20 Drops Clary Sage
10 Drops Cypress
10 Drops Orange
25 Drops Carrier

Happy Ending
20 Drops Joy
15 Drops Lime
10 Drops Cypress
25 Drops Carrier

Apply from the inner mid-thigh

to the leg crease

and 2" below the navel

Him

Tarzan Man
20 Drops Hong Kuai
10 Drops Goldenrod
10 Drops Idaho Blue Spruce
5 Drops Black Pepper
25 Drops Carrier

Wake Up Call
20 Drops Idaho Blue Spruce
10 Drops Cypress
5 Drops Rosemary
5 Drops Nutmeg
25 Drops Carrier

Mister Nice Guy
30 Drops Mister
5 Drops Idaho Blue Spruce
5 Drops Cypress

To The Point
Shutran

Edible Blends

Jaws Edible Love Numb

10 Drop Thieves Vitality

10 Drop Clove Vitality

10 Drop Peppermint Vitality

1 Tablespoon Solid Coconut Oil

5 drops Olive Oil

1/4 teaspoon Agave

Lightly warm the coconut until it melts. Stir in the olive oil and aguave. Stir in the Thieves, Clove and Peppermint. Cool in fridge and use your thumb and apply to the roof of your mouth. Adjust oils as needed to gently numb the back of the throat.

Coco-lime Edible Love Serum

1/2 Teaspoon Beeswax

3 Teapoons Unrefined Solid Coconut Oil

1 Teaspoon Grapeseed Oil

1/2 Teaspoon Coconut Cream

1/2 Teaspoon Agave

25 Drops Lime Vitality

Melt the beeswax and solid coconut oil together. Add the Grapeseed oil, coconut cream, and aguave. Add Lime. Cool and have yourself a tropical party. It's lick-a-licious.

Lucy's Skinamint Edible Love Button Butter

This love button butter is made from all natural edible ingredients with a soft pleasing scent, taste, and texture. It is soft enough that it can be pumped from a pump top, or squeezed from a squeeze tube. Makes over half an ounce and I use it in a 1 oz (30 ml) pump top bottle. It should last several months in a nightstand drawer; but as it contains no preservatives, check for freshness each time it's used. Named by Mr. Libido as tasting like "Skinamint", this edible lube will change the way you think about flavored lubes.... no nasty chemical flavor, and it feels AHHH AHHH AHHHH AHmaaaazing on.

1/2 teaspoon Beeswax

3 teaspoons solid coconut oil

3 teaspoons edible Apricot Seed or Grape Seed Oil

1/4 - 1/2 teaspoon Agave

4-5 drops Young Living Peppermint Vitality

8 drops Young Living Grapefruit Vitality

2 drops Young Living Orange Vitality

Melt the Beeswax and coconut oil together, and then add the apricot/grapeseed oil and agave. Allow to cool and add the Peppermint, Grapefruit, and Orange. Store in a pump top bottle or squeeze top bottle.

Vein Diminisher

This amazing topical roller lightens and reduces
leg veins!In a 10ml roller bottle combine:
40 Drops Lemongrass
20 Drops Cypress
10 Drops Helichrysum.
Fill to the top with Cell-lite massage oil or fractionated
coconut oil. Apply to veins 2x daily for a month, then 1x daily
to maintain.

Mr. Libido's Perky Pill

In an empty 00 veggie capsule combine
5-8 Drops Idaho Blue Spruce
3 Drops Goldenrod
2 Drops Nutmeg
10 Drops Olive Oil

He takes 20 minutes before go time.
Can be used daily.

Scar Diminisher

25 Drops Lavender, 25 Drops Frankinsence
25 Drops Fractionated Coconut Oil
Apply topically to stretch marks or scars 2x daily for a month.

Love Button Lubes

Lucy's Sea Man Love Button Stroking Jelly

K. First off - this is hands-down the best love button stroking jelly on the face of the planet. To get it right though, you need to follow directions carefully. It contains pure preserved aloe vera and grape seed oil. 100% pure aloe vera is too liquid for this recipe. And cheap "aloe vera" concoctions are mostly diluted with water and then thickened artificially. That bright blue gel is only a fraction true aloe and is full of artificial colors, preservatives, thickeners and emulsifiers. Yuck.

To get this recipe right, you need a 99% pure aloe vera with minimal natural preservatives like citric acid and minimal natural thickeners like xanthan/xanthan gum / guar gum. The aloe vera I used was Green Leaf Naturals.

You also need an emulsifying agent to keep this recipe together. I use polysorbate 20, because it is a low toxic and easy to find emulsifier that binds the jelly together. So, we're going to add our own polysorbate 20 emulsifier to the 99% natural aloe. I get mine online from lotion-crafters. You can also buy shea butter, beeswax and vegetable glycerin from them.

The Sea Man Love Button Stroking Jelly is slippery and smooth without absorbing too quickly with a look and feel and consistency of.... well... go and make it. You'll get it. Don't freak out. You'll LOVE it.

The recipe has a base which can have many variations depending on which oils you add. The stroking jelly base is:

Sea Man Stroking Jelly Base

2 Teaspoons 99% pure aloe vera gel like Green Leaf Naturals

1 Teaspoon Grape Seed Oil or Sweet Almond Oil

8-10 Drops Polysorbate 20 Emulsifier

1/2 Teaspoon Vegetable Glycerin

1/2 Teaspoon Vitamin E

Then add your oils. The Recipe for Lucy's Original Sea Men Love Button Stroking Jelly is the stroking base above plus:

Lucy's Original

5 Drops Sensation

3 Drops Cypress

3 Drops Orange

2-3 Drops Peppermint

Combine and place in a 10 -15ml bottle - or in a 1 oz pump top dispenser. You are going to DIE. It is SOOOOOO Good.

Variations for the Sea Man Stroking Jelly Base

Fire and Ice:

5 Drops Cypress

3 Drops Light the Fire

3 Drops Orange

1 Drop Peppermint

Hot Nights:

5 Drops Ylang Ylang

3 Drops Tea Tree

3 Drops Black Pepper

2 Drops Orange

Shivers Up Your Spine

5 Drops Clary Sage

3 Drops Peppermint

3 Drops Cypress

2 Drops Lime

Oh Boy Oh Joy

5 Drops Joy

5 Drops Orange

3 Drops Cypress

1 Drop Nutmeg

Slick Lube Love Button Stroking Oil

This love button stroking oil is similar to the stroking jelly, but in a thick oil formula instead of a jelly.

1/2 Teaspoon Refined Shea Butter

3 Teaspoons Grape Seed Oil or Sweet Almond Oil

1/4 teaspoon Vegetable Glycerin

1/4 teaspoon Vitamin E

Melt the Shea Butter and Grapeseed/Almond Oil together. Then add the Vegetable Glycerin and Vitamin E. Cool and add your oils. For Lucy's Original Slick Lube Love Button Stroking Oil add:

Lucy's Original

5 drops Sensation

3 Drops Cypress

3 Drops Orange

2-3 Drops Peppermint

It makes about 15ml or a half ounce and can be stored in a 15ml EO bottle with a dropper top, or in a 1oz / 30ml pump top bottle. Get ready to scream.

Variations You Can Add to Your Stroking Oil Base

Fire and Ice:

5 Drops Cypress

3 Drops Light the Fire

3 Drops Orange

1 Drop Peppermint

Oh Boy Oh Joy

5 Drops Joy

5 Drops Orange

3 Drops Cypress

1 Drop Nutmeg

Hot Nights:

5 Drops Ylang Ylang

3 Drops Tea Tree

3 Drops Black Pepper

2 Drops Orange

Shivers Up Your Spine

5 Drops Clary Sage

3 Drops Peppermint

3 Drops Cypress

2 Drops Lime

Oil Reference Chart

Oil/Serum	Botanical Name	Contains	Topical	Aromatic	Internal
Clary Sage	*Salva clarea*	Clary Sage	*	*	*
Clove	*Syzygium aromaticum*	Clove	*	*	*
Cypress	*Cupressus Sempervirens*	Cypress	*	*	
Dragon Time	*Oil Blend*	Clary Sage, Fennel, Lavender, Marjoram, Yarrow, Jasmine	*	*	
Endoflex	*Oil Blend*	Spearmint, Sage, Geranium, Myrtle Nutmeg, Chamomile, Sesame seed oil	*	*	
Goldenrod	*Solidago canadenis*	Goldenrod	*	*	*
Grapefruit	*Citrus paradisi*	Grapefruit	*	*	*

Dilution	Application	Safety Considerations
1:1	T) Apply 1-2 drops on Vita Flex points or wrists, as needed A) Diffuse or inhale from the bottle I) Consume 1-2 drops diluted with olive oil in a capsule or in 1 tsp honey up to 3x's daily.	Use with caution during pregnancy. Not for children under 2. Avoid during consumption of alcohol.
1:4	T) Apply 1-2 drops on Vita Flex points or wrists, as needed A) Diffuse or inhale from the bottle I) Consume 1 drop diluted with olive oil in a capsule or in 1 tsp honey up to 3x's daily.	Hot oil, dilute generously. Use with caution during pregnancy. May irritate sensitive skin. Natural anti-coagulant. May enhance the effects of blood thinners.
1:1	T) Apply 2-4 drops on Vita Flex points or wrists, as needed. A) Diffuse or inhale from the bottle.	Use with caution during pregnancy; small amounts on occasion and in dilution.
1:1	T) Apply 2-4 drops on Vita Flex points or wrlts as needed. Apply in a hot compress over lower abdomen or back or any area of discomfort. A) Diffuse or inhale from a bottle.	Use with caution during pregnancy; small amounts on occasion and in dilution.
Neat unless sensitive	T) Apply 2-4 drops over lower back, thyroid, kidneys, liver, feet or Vita Flex points. A) Can be diffused by recommended to be used topically.	Sensitive skin may require more dilution. Use with caution if susceptible to epilepsy; small amounts and in dilution. Contains a small amount of sesame seed carrier oil. Not recommended for those with sesame seed allergies.
1:1	T) Apply 2-4 drops on Vita Flex points or wrists as needed. A) Diffuse or inhale from the bottle. I) Consume 1-3 drops diluted with olive oil in a capsule or in 1 tsp honey up to 3x's daily.	
1:1	T) Apply 2-4 drops on Vita Flex points or wrists as needed. A) Diffuse or inhale from the bottle. I) Consume 2-4 drops diluted with olive oll In a capsule or in 1 tsp honey up to 3x's daily	Photosensitive. Avoid direct sunlight after use.

Oil/Serum	Botanical Name	Contains	Topical	Aromatic	Internal
Hong Kuai	*Chamaecyparis formosensis*	Hong Kuai	*	*	
Idaho Blue Spruce	*Picea pungens*	Idaho Blue Spruce	*	*	*
Jasmine	*Jasiminum officinale*	Jasmine	*	*	*
Joy	*Oil Blend*	Bergamot, Ylang Ylang, Geranium, Rosewood, Lemon, Mandarin, Jasmine, Chamomile, Palmarosa, Rose	*	*	
Lady Sclareol	*Oil Blend*	Rosewood, Vetiver, Geranium, Orange, Clary Sage, Ylang Ylang, Sandalwood, Jasmine, Sage Lavender, Idaho Tansy	*	*	
Lime	*Citrus aurantifolia*	Lime	*	*	*
Mister	*Oil Blend*	Sage, Fennel, Lavender, Myrtle, Peppermint, Yarrow	*	*	

Dilution	Application	Safety Considerations
1:1	T) Apply 2-4 drops on Vita Flex points, forehead, back of neck or outside of ear, as needed. A) Diffuse or inhale from the bottle	Avoid during pregnancy. Keep out of reach of children.
Neat unless sensitive	T) Apply 2-4 drops on Vita Flex points or wrists, as needed. A) Diffuse or inhale from the bottle. I) Consume 3-8 drops diluted with olive oil, in capsule or in 1 tsp honey 1x daily.	
Neat unless sensitive	T) Apply 2-4 drops on Vita Flex points or wrists, as needed. A) Diffuse or inhale from the bottle. I) Consume 1-3 drops diluted with olive oil, in capsule or in 1 tsp honey up to 3x's daily.	
1:1	T) Apply 2-4 drops over the heart, thymus, temples or wrists, as needed. A) Diffuse or inhale from the bottle.	Citrus Oils contained in this blend are photosensitive. Avoid direct sunlight after use.
Neat unless sensitive	T) Apply 2-4 drops on the clavicle notch, wrists, and ankles daily or as needed. A) Diffuse or inhale from the bottle.	Use with caution during pregnancy: small amounts on occasion and in dilution. Not for children under 2.
1:1	T) Apply 1-2 drops on Vita Flex points or wrists, as needed. A) Diffuse or inhale from the bottle. I) Consume 2-4 drops diluted with olive oil in a capsule or in 1 tsp honey up to 3x's daily.	Photosensitive. Avoid direct sunlight after use.
Neat unless sensitive	T) Apply 2-4 drops on Vita Flex points, lower pelvis or wrists as needed. Use in a hot compress. A) Diffuse or inhale from the bottle.	Avoid during pregnancy. Use with caution if susceptible to epilepsy: small amounts and in dilution. Contains a small amount of Sesame Seed carrier oil. Not recommended for sesame seed allergies.

Oil/Serum	Botanical Name	Contains	Topical	Aromatic	Internal
Nutmeg	*Myristica fragrans*	Nutmeg	*	*	*
Orange	*Citrus aurantium*	Orange	*	*	*
Pepper, black	*Piper nigrum*	Black Pepper	*	*	*
Peppermint	*Mentha piperita*	Peppermint	*	*	*
Progessence Plus Serum	*Oil Serum*	Copaiba, Cedarwood, Sacred Frankincense, Coconut oil, Bergamot, Peppermint, Rosewood, Wild Yam Extract sourced Progesterone, Clove, Vitamin E	*		
Sandalwood	*Santalum album*	Sandalwood	*	*	*
Sclaressence	*Oil Blend*	Clary Sage, Peppermint, Sage Lavender, Fennel	*		*

Dilution	Application	Safety Considerations
1:2	T) Apply 1-2 drops on Vita Flex points or wrists, as needed. A) Diffuse or inhale from the bottle. I) Consume 1-2 drops diluted with olive oil in a capsule or in 1 tsp honey up to 3x's daily.	Not for children under 6. Not for use by people with epilepsy: small amounts and in dilution. Use with caution during pregnancy. Do not over-use or exceed 3 undiluted drops at once.
1:1	T) Apply 2-3 drops on Vita Flex points or wrists, as needed. A) Diffuse or inhale from the bottle. I) Consume 1-3 drops diluted with olive oil in a capsule or in 1 tsp honey up to 3x's daily.	Photosensitive. Avoid direct sunlight after use.
1:1	T) Apply 2-4 drops on Vita Flex points or wrists as needed. A) Diffuse or inhale from the bottle. I) Consume 1-3 drops diluted with olive oil in a capsule or in 1 tsp honey up to 3x's daily.	Use with greater dilution in children under 6. May feel warm to sensitive skin.
1:2	T) Apply 1-2 drops on abdomen, temples, wrists, or Vita Flex points, as needed. A) diffuse or inhale from the bottle. I) Consume 1-3 drops diluted with olive oil in a capsule of 1 tsp honey up to 3x's daily.	Avoid use on the abdominal area during pregnancy. Use with caution and with greater dilution with children. May reduce milk supply in some nursing mothers.
Neat unless sensitive	T) Apply 2-4 drops over the carotid arteries, on the neck and/or along the forearms. Use 1-2 times daily or as needed on the temples, for menstrual headaches. Application at night may aid sleep.	Use under the supervision of a doctor if you have a genetic disorder called Factor V Leiden. Use with caution when taking contraceptives that contain progesterone or prescribed progestin's. May cause spotting or a change in menstrual cycle with starting. See Progessence Plus FAQ for more details.
Neat unless sensitive	T) Apply 1-2 drops on Vita Flex points or wrists, as needed. A) Diffuse or inhale from the bottle. I) Consume 1-2 drops diluted, with olive oil in a capsule or in 1 tsp honey.	
Neat unless sensitive	T) Apply on ankles and wrists I) Consume 1-10 drops in a capsule with olive oil. Start with 1 drop and increase as needed, up to 20 drops daily.	Not recommended for children.

Oil/Serum	Botanical Name	Contains	Topical	Aromatic	Internal
Sensation	*Oil blend*	Rosewood, Ylang Ylang, Jasmine	*	*	
Shutran	*Oil blend*	Idaho Blue Spruce, Ocotea, Ylang Ylang, Hinoki, Coriander, Davana, Lavender, Cedarwood, Lemon, Northern Lights Black Spruce	*	*	
Tea Tree	*Melaleuca alternifoli*	Tea Tree	*	*	*
Theives	*Oil Blend*	Clove, Lemon, Cinnamon Bark, Eucalyptus Radiata, Rosemary	*	*	*
Valor	*Oil blend*	Black Spruce, Rosewood, Blue Tansy, Frankincense	*	*	
Ylang Ylang	*Cananga odorata*	Ylang Ylang	*	*	*

Dilution	Application	Safety Considerations
Neat unless sensitive	T) Apply 2-4 drops on Vita Flex points or wrists, as needed. A) Diffuse or inhale from bottle	
Neat unless sensitive	T) Apply 2-4 drops daily to Vita Flex points, neck or wrists. A) Diffuse or inhale from bottle.	Not recommended when you don't have the time to dramatically increase sex frequency. I just included that to see if you read safety information. Which you should...
1:1	T) Apply 2-4 drops on Vita Flex points or wrists, as needed. A) Diffuse or inhale from the bottle. I) Consume 1 drop diluted with olive oil in a capsule or in 1 tsp honey 1x daily.	Use with greater dilution in children under 6. May feel warm to sensitive skin.
1:2	T) Apply 2-4 drops on Vita Flex points or wrists, as needed. A) Diffuse or inhale from the bottle. I) Consume 2-4 drops diluted with olive oil in a capsule or in 1 tsp honey up to 3x's daily.	Hot oil so dilute generously. Use with greater dilution with children under 6 or during pregnancy.
Neat unless sensitive	T) Apply 2-4 drops on Vita Flex points, wrists, heart, throat and thymus, as needed. Recommended on the bottom of the feet. A) Diffuse or inhale from the bottle	Contains a small amount of almond carrier oil. Not recommended for those with almond allergies.
1:1	T) Apply 2-4 drops on Vita Flex points, thymus, or wrists, as needed. A) Diffuse or inhale from the bottle. I) Consume 1 drop, diluted with olive oil in a capsule or in 1 tsp honey 1x daily.	Use with greater dilution for sensitive skin.

Dr. Dan Purser, M.D.

Answers to

Frequently asked questions about Progessence Plus and their answers from Dr. Purser

Here are just some of the questions we've received:

Is Progessence Plus® safe to take? Yes. It's just that simple. It contains a tiny amount of a biologically identical (to humans) hormone called progesterone that is not only safe, but incredibly beneficial to women. Natural progesterone has no long-term problems associated with it – even at high doses.

Are natural hormones safe to take? Yes, they are very safe to take. Studies have shown that synthetic hormones may have health risks that may exceed the benefits of HRT. A woman's body has trouble assimilating synthetic hormones effectively and the side effects that result are often much worse than the original problems being treated.

Why is there a statement about causing cancer on the package? This is an outdated statement which is required by law, in California. Proposition 65 is placed on anything brought into the state of California that contains hormones. Unfortunately, the law does not differentiate between synthetic and natural hormones. Young Living has a Progessence cream, which also carries the required Prop 65 statement on the tube. This is because synthetic medroxyprogesterone acetate (which is found in so many products made for women) along with the synthetics in the various birth control pills, have all been shown to cause cancer. Research has proven that natural human progesterone does not.

Here is Young Living's official statement about the Warning on the label:

—There is no cancer causing agents in Progessence Plus®. This statement is due to an outdated California law that actually refers to the cancer known to be caused by the synthetic medroxyprogesterone acetate (MPA as in the drug Provera) which has been shown in a number of studies to cause breast cancer. But MPA is not the human P4 or bio- identical progesterone made from natural yam products that we used in Progessence Plus® – the generic chemical names are just similar. But the law is poorly written and mistakenly refers to any hormone as cancer causing when no naturally occurring human hormone has been associated with any cancer ever (not even estradiol – CEE has but no human 17-beta- estradiol). Human progesterone (even the compounded version like in Progessence Plus®) actually reduces breast and ovarian cancer risk (and reduces a lot of other risks such as CAD, stroke, DVT, etc). This can all be verified by searching on PubMed. If you live in California please lobby for the change of this law. Thank you for the great question.

Does this mean I won't get cancer now that I'm using Progessence Plus®? No, it can and in some cases, will still happen. We just hope it reduces your risk. Let me be clear – Progessence Plus® and progesterone will not cure you of cancer, nor do I want to give you any idea that it will. Medically & legally, I am ethically bound to say that if you indeed have cancer please follow the instructions of your allopathic (western) physicians (or physicians of your choosing) and have the proper surgeries or therapies. I have found that faith can also do marvelous things and I pray for those of you whose lives have been affected by cancer. God bless you.

I take birth control pills (or shots) and wonder why I can't take the Progessence Plus®? If or when you develop blood clots or breast cancer from the synthetics we don't want Progessence Plus® to be associated in any way or on the radar screen of possible causes when your attorney is looking for culprits. Natural progesterone does not cause clots or breast cancer, period. Research has proven that synthetics are cancer causing and if you are using synthetics, it would be too easy for doctors to point the blame at the natural product. The safe and 100% natural human progesterone reduces your risks of clots, strokes, heart attacks and cools your arteries besides.

I've had breast cancer and my doctor says not to take any hormones – why? Because synthetic hormones have been associated with breast cancer and as all hormones can sometimes be lumped into the same category, this opinion of staying away from hormones has tainted natural hormones as well (There is no data that supports the connection between synthetic and natural hormones).

This is the like the Proposition 65 Statement law required in California where they combine all of the hormones in one category, then they make a broad sweeping and inaccurate statement about them. They are not even remotely similar. However; you should still talk to your doctor and get their approval to use Progessence Plus® if you have any questions about it.

If my doctor says not to take Progessence Plus®, what should I do?

Hopefully, your doctor is trained in preventive medicine, endocrinology, gynecology, or is well versed in natural and modern methods of prevention. Today there is so much information available about hormones that your doctor should be able to provide you with a well researched reason to avoid it. I would suggest you seek a second opinion. But always listen to your doctor FIRST.

I've had progesterone receptor (PR+) positive breast cancer; can I take Progessence Plus®? Again, please talk to your personal physician first. If you were my patient, I would say that because of your experience with cancer, that it is even more reason to use a natural progesterone product. Research continues to prove that natural or human progesterone will connect to that progesterone receptor and cause apoptosis (see my book on Progesterone for more details) or —destruction‖ of the cell.

I have endometriosis – will Progessence Plus® be safe for me to take? Progessence Plus® is not only safe but from may studies we know progesterone will probably help your endometriosis maybe even dramatically reduce your symptoms.

I am 18 and have severe PMS – is Progessence Plus® safe to take? Progessence Plus® is not only safe, but we know from lots of studies that progesterone will probably help your PMS. We've found that it usually does help.

I have menstrual migraines -- is Progessence Plus® safe to take? Yes -- research has shown the positive effect natural progesterone has on migraine headaches.

I've had a hysterectomy so why would I take Progessence Plus®? Lack of progesterone can occur whether your ovaries are there or not – and as a woman you need a sufficient amount of progesterone to balance your hormones.

I've had blood clots from birth control pills – is Progessence Plus® safe to take? Synthetic progestins are known to cause clots, while human (natural) progesterone has been shown in a number of studies to not cause clots. I would consult with your physician to be sure, but I believe that you can safely take Progessence Plus® without increasing your risk of more blood clots.

I've had a stroke/heart attack -- is Progessence Plus® safe to take? Synthetic progestins are known to cause strokes or heart attacks (vascular disease), while human (natural) progesterone has been shown in a number of studies to reduce vascular inflammation and heart attacks/strokes. I believe that you are safe to use Progessence Plus®, but I would consult with your doctor if you have any concerns.

I have insomnia -- is Progessence Plus® safe to take? Yes, progesterone has been shown to cause somnolence (sleepiness) in women and you could find yourself sleeping deeper when using it.

I have hot flashes/night sweats -- can Progessence Plus® help? Yes, lack of progesterone has been shown to stop these 98% of the time. (You might try the Young Living product, FemiGen, to take care of the other 2% -- it increases estrone.)

I have no libido – will Progessence Plus® make this worse? No, research has shown that using progesterone should improve libido – so go ahead and try some, but warn your honey first!

Can Progessence Plus® be taken with thyroid medications? Absolutely! And they do not cross react.

I have had a breast removed, can I use Progessence Plus®? What if I am currently being treated for breast cancer? Always ask your doctor first before adding anything to your routine, but we, of course, would encourage you to use Progessence Plus® (as long as they approve).

Is Progessence Plus® safe for breast cancer survivors taking tamoxifen? Ask your doctor of course, but yes, we believe so.

What are the implications of using Progessence Plus® on MS patients? The implications are really good—and so I suggest taking more. I know from the literature and our experiences that the top teaching hospitals advise all kind of hormones for their patients (like testosterone) and progesterone because it is thought to be quite beneficial in remyelinating nerves. It's unfortunate that a lot of docs don't read the research or literature, but instead let drug companies influence their opinions on medical issues.

How would you recommend taking this serum? Begin with just a drop on your neck or the hairless part of your arm each night and let your body adjust to the intake of progesterone. You can increase the amount as you feel the need, but I would advise you to start with a small amount and increase it over time. Remember that every woman will react differently to the increased progesterone levels in her body, so be aware that you may have some kind of reaction too. Sometimes women using Progessence Plus® experience an increase in hot flashes and that sometimes indicates an increase in application of Progessence Plus® is needed before they subside.

How should menopausal women use this serum? Probably daily, I suggest that they rub it on their neck or hairless parts of their forearms.

Is there a maximum amount a day that I should use? Follow what the instructions on the bottle say however; I say take as much as you feel that you need. (Remember that your serum progesterone levels can get 400X higher with pregnancy.)

How many milligrams (mg) of progesterone are in a drop of Progessence Plus®? Well, Progessence Plus® has less than 15 mg per ml of progesterone (about 14.2 or so – just about the max allowed by the FDA) but the secret is in the quality of the progesterone we used. One milliliter (ml) has about 30 drops total in it and so one drop has about 0.5-1.0 mg of progesterone. All of this may be technical talk and is meaningless when compared to the quality of this product and absorption properties. There are a number of poor quality progesterone's out there for oral or sublingual use, and thankfully we will never keep company with any of them. What we do know is that as you are testing this, your body will appreciate your daily applications.

Can Progessence Plus® replace my oral or sublingual progesterone completely? Possibly but it's according to the quality and amount of the progesterone that you're taking at night. Remember to check with your doctor before changing over. Progessence Plus® is certainly good to take in addition to sublingual or oral progesterone.

Why do I get a headache whenever I use Progessence Plus®? This is a little uncommon but it can occur, especially if you have a lot of vascular inflammation – it's kind of a way your blood vessels fight back against the relaxation and reduction in inflammation going on after you apply Progessence Plus®. If you have this symptom then only apply small amounts before bed and build up slowly over a matter of months.

My high cholesterol problem went away (or improved) when I used Progessence Plus® – my doctor is mystified by this – what happened? We know from a number of good studies that in women increasing progesterone often causes a drop in cholesterol levels sometimes returning them back to normal. It's a cool benefit (literally for your arteries) and is one of the reasons why progesterone has been shown to reduce the risk of stroke and heart attacks in women.

Can I use Progessence Plus® with Depo-Provera? These synthetic hormones cause vascular inflammation and thus blood clots and strokes/heart attacks – human or natural progesterone does not. So when or if you have these side effects we do not want our wonderful Progessence Plus® being associated with these in any way shape or

form – that's all. We're being protective of our product and don't want to be colored with the same brush as the synthetics.

Can men use Progessence Plus® for any reason? NO! We get asked this all the time so let me answer it again – HECK NO! It causes a decrease in libido and vascular inflammation (mild) in men – so best to be avoided by men.

I get up every morning and apply my Progessence Plus® and then I feel dizzy all morning – why? Progesterone lowers blood pressure (by relaxing arteries) – this is why, if you have just started using Progessence Plus® and have had years of low progesterone you should not use Progessence Plus® in the morning (start at night until your body gets used to it again). It also makes some women very sleepy so again another reason to take before bed. After you're used to it again for a while THAN you can start adding it in the morning.

Is Progessence Plus® safe to use with my regular BHRT (Bio-identical Hormone Replacement Therapy)? Absolutely and may help with your regular BHRT (can't hurt) but ask your doctor before you do this.

Is Progessence Plus® safe to use, with synthetic progesterone (sic – progestins)? Yes but we'd prefer you didn't because, again, we don't want Progessence Plus® caught in the blame game when women start having the blood clots, strokes, breast cancer and other side effects that are common from the synthetics.

Can Progessence Plus® replace my oral/sublingual progesterone in my regular BHRT (Bio-identical Hormone Replacement Therapy)? Possibly – in my experience, most of the compounded hormones out there, are not of a very good quality. But if curious, get your doctor to check levels before and after. And make sure they approve this first.

Is Progessence Plus® safe to take with DHEA or Young Living products containing DHEA? Sure, why not? These are not mutually exclusive in any way and both are natural hormones produced in your body so they work together – remember though, do not take DHEA if you have a personal breast cancer risk factor.

Will Progessence Plus® balance my estrogen dominance issue? The natural Progessence in Progessence Plus® should help or may actually do it if it's not too severe an imbalance. If I have high estrogen levels, how can I lower my levels of estrogen? You don't try to lower estrogen levels in estrogen dominance, but instead you raise your progesterone level to balance it out. Use Progessence Plus® to do this and if you would have any questions, check with your doctor when balancing your hormones.

Is Progessence Plus® safe with any cancer? Sure, why not? It's a natural hormone not associated with causation of any cancer (though the lack of progesterone has been associated with a higher risk of a number of cancers). Remember though to talk to your doctor first.

Is Progessence Plus® safe with prolactinomas and adenomas of the pituitary? Yes, sure, why not? There's no connection between the two at all. If a woman makes progesterone in her ovaries and develops a pituitary tumor or brain tumor, doctors don't start ripping out ovaries usually (hopefully never). So it's safe – but make sure you talk to your doctor first.

I have endometriosis and my doctor wants to do a hysterectomy – in light of this is Progessence Plus® safe to take? Yes. They are taking out the uterus probably because with endometriosis you're bleeding and are miserable.

I believe that they're just doing the best they can to try to help. I disagree with encouraging women to have hysterectomies. I personally like to treat endometriosis with lots of progesterone until symptoms resolve, but I'm not your doctor so talk to them first.

I have really high blood pressure that is difficult to treat – is Progessence Plus® safe to take? I have received hundreds of emails from women saying —WOW - my blood pressure has gone way down‖ and that is what the medical studies show as well. In almost every study I have read, the women taking progesterone have experienced lower blood pressure. So yes, take it and chances are very good that you will have lower blood pressure sometime soon.

I have heavy menstrual bleeding, is Progessence Plus® safe to take in this situation? Yes, progesterone has been shown to reduce crazy heavy bleeding – this is why gynecologists use synthetic birth control pills to control this kind of periodic bleeding, so try the natural progesterone instead – safer and equally beneficial results.

My daughter has menstrual migraines, should she try cycling Progessence Plus® to see if this assists? Sure, it may help. When she has signs or symptoms just try a drop on her neck (over her carotids) – you'll see if it gives her some relief.

My daughter is 11 and complains of stomach aches low down in her abdomen once a month – I think she's almost ready to start her cycles – can I use Progessence Plus® with her? Sure – these are probably early or pre-menarche PMS symptoms – so give her a little to see if she benefits.

My doctor says I have uterine polyps/fibroids/ovarian cysts – can I use Progessence Plus®? Uterine polyps/fibroids/ovarian cysts have all been shown to be caused by low levels of progesterone over long periods of time – so it does not hurt to take Progessence Plus® now.

Does taking Progessence Plus® reduce my own production of progesterone? No, no, no. Never! Topical progesterone does not cause negative feedback loop suppression like birth control pills cause. The serum just adds to your levels.

How do I know I really need Progessence Plus®? You can get levels checked -- 99% of women we checked at the Young Living International Grand Convention of 2010 in Salt Lake City effectively had zero levels (<0.20 ng/ml) of progesterone in their blood – no matter what their age. This was appalling. Plus if you have symptoms of low progesterone (hot flashes, night sweats, migraines, loss of libido, depression, etc) you may benefit.

How does Progessence Plus® compare to oral or sublingual progesterone my doctor gave me? This is a common question we've gotten – they don't really or it's kind of like comparing apples to peanuts – there's no way other than by the way you feel and following blood levels can you tell for sure. Maybe your progesterone you're using is not very well micronized or maybe it's very well micronized and you're running optimized levels – either way there's no way of knowing without blood levels or symptom alleviation.

Does Progessence Plus® help women get pregnant? Anything that increases progesterone levels in pre-menopausal women who have chronically low progesterone levels may benefit attempts to get pregnant. We don't know for sure but our guess it might indeed.

Is Progessence Plus® safe to take with other medications besides BCPs? Always ask your doctor but we'd say yes. It's a just a little low dose topical progesterone in Vitamin E (with a few critical essential oils) so we'd say sure – no problem. But please ask your doctor first.

Which facilities do you recommend using to get my levels tested? You may download my Purser Preferred Lab Solutions PDF for free at www.drpurser.com. It will give you info on my preferred labs and where your levels should be.

Disclamer: The information contained in this FAQ is intended for educational purposes only. It is not intended to substitute for medical care or to prescribe treatment for any specific health condition. Dr. Dan Purser, M.D. and Young Living assume no responsibility to or liability for any person or group for any loss, damage, or injury resulting from the use or misuse of any information herein.

Notes

All About Lucy

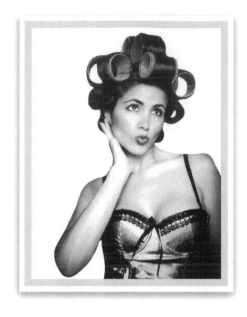

Lucy Libido is the creator of the ever popular Facebook Class
Lucy Libido Says… There's an Oil for THAT

You can find her on Facebook through her friend page
"Lucy Li Bido" or through her fan page "Lucy Libido"
You can also follow her on Instagram at "lucylibido"

To order more copies of this book, visit us at

www.lucylibido.com

For special discounts on bulk orders or to arrange for Lucy to
speak at your next event, email lucy@lucylibido.com

Need to order oils? Amazon is a great place to buy books. It
is NOT a safe place to order oils. Contact your enroller or
the person who gave you this book. They will show you how
to have your oils shipped directly from the farm to your door.
Don't have an oil guru yet? Message Lucy through Facebook
or email lucy@lucylibido.com for a proper referral.

Made in the USA
San Bernardino, CA
30 January 2017